Pharmacy Museums
and Historical Collections

A GUIDE TO PHARMACY MUSEUMS AND HISTORICAL COLLECTIONS IN THE UNITED STATES AND CANADA

by

George Griffenhagen

Ernst W. Stieb

Beth D. Fisher

American Institute of the History of Pharmacy
Madison, Wisconsin
1999

I.S.B.N. 0-931292-34-4

Publication No. 18 (New Series)
Gregory J. Higby and Elaine C. Stroud, General Editors

Cover: Hooks American Drugstore Museum, located in Indianapolis, Indiana.

Contents

Introduction

The artistic drug jars and the mysterious concoctions produced in the pharmacy have always attracted public attention. Hence, it is not surprising that for centuries museums have collected and exhibited the individual curiosities of the apothecary shop. In fact, as early as the seventeenth century, the Dresden Museum in Germany displayed the restoration of a complete apothecary shop.

By 1931, there were so many European museums with apothecary shop restorations and pharmaceutical history exhibits that Josef Anton Häfliger of Basel, Switzerland, published a listing of 230 public and private pharmaceutico-historical collections.[1]

The first collection of pharmaceutical artifacts in the United States was organized by the Philadelphia College of Pharmacy shortly after its founding in 1821.[2] The earliest attempt in this country to preserve an entire section of a pharmacy was made by the Historical Society of Newport, Rhode Island; in 1884, the Society secured the show window from *Charles Feke's Apothecary Shop* established in Newport in 1796, and installed it outside their building directly over the entrance.[3]

In 1897, the Wisconsin Pharmaceutical Association appointed a Historical Committee, with Edward Kremers as chairman, to collect state and local historical material of celebrate the 50th anniversary of Wisconsin statehood. For a number of years thereafter the students and faculty of the University of Wisconsin School of Pharmacy collected pharmaceutical antiques from all over the state which was assembled and installed in the fall of 1913 as a *Pioneer Drug Store* restoration at the State Historical Society of Wisconsin.[4]

In the meantime, the equipment and part of the fixtures of the *Glentworth Apothecary Shop* of Philadelphia were restored by the Philadelphia College of Pharmacy and exhibited in the Hall of Horticultural Society for the 1902 American Pharmaceutical Association semi-centennial annual meeting.[5] The APhA 1902 *Catalogue of the Historical Exhibition* described the restoration as "Ye Olde Apothecary -- portions of a Philadelphia drug store as it appeared in the early part of the nineteenth century."

In his 1903 report to the APhA Section on Historical Pharmacy, Edward Kremers proposed the formation of a committee to organize collections representing a drugstore of the period 1848 to 1898 in "each State of the Union and each province of Canada."[6]

Perhaps as a result of this appeal, the Essex Institute of Salem, Massachusetts, opened for exhibition an old New England apothecary shop restoration in 1913; the Charleston Museum in South Carolina installed the fixtures and equipment of *Apothecaries Hall* in 1921;[7] and the *Hugh Mercer Apothecary Shop* in Fredericksburg, Virginia, was restored and opened for exhibition in 1928.[8] The American Pharmaceutical Association cooperated in the arrangement of the pharmacy exhibits at the 1933-1934 *Chicago Century of Progress Exposition*, which included the pharmacy restoration of Chicago's *Philo Carpenter Drug Store*. Also in 1933, the *Stabler-Leadbeater Apothecary Shop* of Alexandria, Virginia, was sold under the auctioneer's gavel with the understanding that the American Pharmaceutical Association would assure its reopening as a permanent pharmacy museum, which took place in 1939.[9]

From April 1953 to August 1954, the *Journal of the American Pharmaceutical Association* published a series of monographs entitled "Early American Pharmacies." The series was reprinted in 1955 as a pictorial catalog of apothecary shop restorations which are on exhibition in the United States.[10] The following year, the American Institute of the History of Pharmacy (AIHP) published a handbook by George Griffenhagen entitled *Pharmacy Museums* which featured an annotated list of pharmacy museums worldwide.[11]

Published by AIHP in 1957, *American Pharmacy's Historical Collections*, an eight-page brochure by Griffenhagen, was described by Glenn Sonnedecker as "a pocket companion for the pharmacist-traveler, and for others who would find diversion or instruction in the tangible remains of pharmacy's past."[12]

By 1963, all previous publications were out-of-print, so an international guide of pharmacy museums was incorporated into Glenn Sonnedecker's revision of *Kremers and Urdang's History of Pharmacy*,[13] and the AIHP pamphlet was revised in 1965 by George Griffenhagen and Cleo Sonnedecker.[14]

Sami K. Hamarneh assumed responsibility in 1972 for authoring the third revision of the AIHP guide to pharmacy museums now titled *Pharmacy Museums in the U.S.A.*[15] The same year, Hamarneh authored an equally useful book entitled *Temples of the Muses and a History of Pharmacy Museums*.[16]

The AIHP guidebook of pharmacy museums was expanded in 1981 to include those in Canada as well as in the United States. Entitled *Pharmacy Museum and Historical Collections on Public View in the United States and Canada*, the guidebook was co-authored by Sami K. Hamarneh and Ernst W. Stieb of Canada.[17]

This AIHP guidebook of pharmacy museums in Canada and in the United States, entitled *Pharmacy Museums and Historical Collections in the United States and Canada,* was updated in 1988. Co-authored by Griffenhagen and Stieb, this 92-page book also included a review of "Historical Pharmacy Markers" and a subject index.[18]

Like the 1988 edition, this revised guidebook has been arranged in the following order: Museums in the United States are described in monographs listed in alphabetical order by state (including the District of Columbia, Puerto Rico, and the Virgin Islands) and then alphabetically by city. These are followed by monographs of Canadian museums in alphabetical order by province and then by city. They have been edited by Griffenhagen, Stieb and Fisher with the invaluable assistance of Gregory J. Higby and Elaine C. Stroud.

In accordance with American custom and usage, the terms apothecary shop, pharmacy, and drugstore are used synonymously as they relate to the exhibitions described in the individual monographs.

Days and hours of opening, as well as admission fees, are listed when known. To save space, the monographs do not include the days that the museums are closed (i.e., Thanksgiving, Christmas, and New Year's Day). Since all of these are subject to change, it is advisable to check with the museum prior to embarking on a special side trip; or make special arrangements by telephone or by letter with the curator before a visit.

The co-authors hope that this guidebook will prove to be as useful as its predecessors, and believe that the reader/user will discover -- as previously suggested by Glenn Sonnedecker -- that the "apothecary's lore linked to the nostalgic, the curious, and the beautiful, appeals as strongly to the layman as it does to the pharmacist." As with prior editions, the co-authors urge readers/users to let the American Institute of the History of Pharmacy know of any noteworthy public collections in the United States or Canada that may have escaped our attention.

George Griffenhagen

References

1. Josef Anton Häfliger, *Pharmazeutische Altertumskunde*, B. Wepf & Cie., Basel, Switzerland, 1931.
2. Joseph W. England, *The First Century of the Philadelphia College of Pharmacy*, Philadelphia, 1922.
3. "Dr. William Hunter of Newport," *Annals of Surgery*, January 1935; and "My Favorite Druggist," *Cosmopolitan*, November 1951.
4. *The Pioneer Drug Store*, State Historical Society of Wisconsin, June 1930. See also *Pharmaceutical Era*, 50:45, 1917; and *Tile and Till*, 19:86, 1933.
5. *Catalogue of the Historical Exhibition, Semi-Centennial Anniversary of the American Pharmaceutical Association*, September 8-13, 1902.
6. Edward Kremers, *Proceedings of the American Pharmaceutical Association*, 51:541, 1903.
7. John Bennett, *Apothecaries' Hall*, Charleston Museum, Charleston, South Carolina, 1923.
8. J.M. Waterman, *With Sword and Lancet*, Garrett and Massie, Richmond, Virginia, 1941. See also *Journal of the American Pharmaceutical Association, Practical Pharmacy Edition*, 2:61, 1941.
9. *Journal of the American Pharmaceutical Association*, 22:705, 1933; Ibid., 23:1137, 1934.
10. George Griffenhagen, *Early American Pharmacies*, American Pharmaceutical Association, Washington, DC, 1955.
11. George Griffenhagen, *Pharmacy Museums*, American Institute of the History of Pharmacy, Madison, Wisconsin, 1956.
12. George Griffenhagen, *American Pharmacy's Historical Collections*, American Institute of the History of Pharmacy, Madison, Wisconsin, n.d. [1957].
13. Glenn Sonnedecker, *Kremers and Urdang's History of Pharmacy*, Third Edition, J.B. Lippincott, 1963, pp. 384-395. The "International List of Pharmacy Museums" was updated and again published in Glenn Sonnedecker's Fourth Edition of *Kremers and Urdang's History of Pharmacy*, J.B. Lippincott, 1976, pp. 396-417.
14. George Griffenhagen and Cleo Sonnedecker, *American Pharmacy's Historical Collections*, American Institute of the History of Pharmacy, Madison, Wisconsin, 1965.
15. Sami K. Hamarneh, *Pharmacy Museums U.S.A.*, American Institute of the History of Pharmacy, Madison, Wisconsin, 1972.
16. Sami K. Hamarneh, *Temples of the Muses and a History of Pharmacy Museums*, The Naito Foundation, Tokyo, Japan, 1972.
17. Sami K. Hamarneh and Ernst W. Stieb, *Pharmacy Museums and Historical Collections on Public View in the United States and Canada*, American Institute of the History of Pharmacy, Madison, Wisconsin, in cooperation with the Smithsonian Institution, Washington, DC., 1981.
18. George Griffenhagen and Ernst W. Stieb, *Pharmacy Museums and Historical Collections in the United States and Canada*, American Institute of the History of Pharmacy, Madison, Wisconsin, 1988.

1906

Annual Price List

WHITALL TATUM COMPANY

MANUFACTURERS OF

DRUGGISTS', CHEMISTS', and PERFUMERS'

GLASSWARE

MANUFACTURERS, IMPORTERS, AND JOBBERS OF

DRUGGISTS' SUNDRIES

PHILADELPHIA
410-416 RACE STREET
P. O. BOX 1633

NEW YORK
46 & 48 BARCLAY STREET
P. O. BOX 1866

BOSTON
91 WASHINGTON STREET NORTH

SAN FRANCISCO
45 STEVENSON STREET

SYDNEY, N. S. W.
12 BARRACK STREET

SAMPLES OF OUR GOODS CAN BE SEEN AT OUR CHICAGO SAMPLE ROOM, 196 EAST RANDOLPH STREET

FACTORIES: MILLVILLE, N. J.

Illustrations of druggists' sundries from the Whitall Tatum Company Catalog of 1906.

Pharmacy Museums and Historical Collections in the United States

ALABAMA

BIRMINGHAM

Alabama Museum of Health Science
Lister Hill Library of the Health Sciences
University of Alabama at Birmingham
1700 University Boulevard
University Station, AL 35294-0013
(205) 934-4475

Managed by the University of Alabama at Birmingham.
Michael Flannery, executive director.

Monday - Friday 8:00 a.m. - 5:00 p.m.

Admission - free

A large hall includes exhibitions on pharmaceutical tools, drug bottles, medical and dental equipment, nursing and ophthalmological artifacts, together with documents, photographs, memorabilia, and archival material related to the health professions in the state of Alabama. In an adjacent hall is the Lawrence Reynolds Historical Library, which includes rare books and archives.

JACKSONVILLE

Dr. J. C. Francis Medical Museum
100 Gayle Street
Jacksonville, AL 36265
(256) 435-7611, ext. 8

Managed by the State of Alabama Historical Commission, 468 S. Perry Street, Montgomery, AL 36130-0900, (334) 242-3184 ext. 248.

Open by appointment only.

Admission - free

The museum and grounds are owned by the Alabama State Historical Commission. The museum was opened to the public on March 21, 1974, when a marker in memory of Dr. J.C. Francis was unveiled by his great-grandson.

The restored structure consists of two rooms, an apothecary shop in front leading into a physician's office in the rear. The building was constructed about 1850 and was occupied by Dr. Francis for almost forty of his fifty-four years of practice as a family physician in Jacksonville. On display are apothecary jars and medicine bottles, a plantation first-aid kit, surgical instruments, and various medication containers similar to those used or dispensed to clients more than a century ago. In addition, other period furnishings, scales, apothecary tools, journals, and books of the 1820s to the 1870s are exhibited.

MOBILE

Mobile Medical Museum
1504 Springhill Avenue
Mobile, AL 36604
(334) 434-5055

Owned by Friends of the Mobile Medical Museum.
Patsy Starkey, administrator.

Monday - Friday 8:00 a.m. - 5:00 p.m.

Admission - free

Heritage collection of artifacts in a hands-on museum with interactive health education emphasis. In the fall of 1999, the museum will move to 355 Government Street. The new museum will include partnerships with the Drug Education Council, the Medical Society of Mobil County; the Retired Nurses Association; and the Alliance to the Medical Society with Camp Rap-A-Hope for children with cancer. The museum has an extensive collection of old Mobile drugstore bottles. Dr. Sam Eichold, founder of the museum, is the son of the first wholesale druggist in the State of Alabama (Mobile Drug Company).

HORN SPOONS. Long Handle.

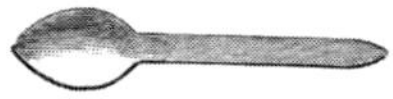

No.	Per doz.	No.	Per doz.
⅛.	$1 00	3.	$1 60
¼.	1 00	4.	2 15
1.	1 10	6.	2 50
2.	1 35	7.	3 50

Montgomery

Alabama Pharmacy Association
1211 Carmichael Way
Montgomery, AL 36106-3672
(334) 271-4222

Owned and operated by the Alabama Pharmacist Association. David L. Laven, executive director.

E-mail DLaven@aparx.org

Monday - Friday 8:00 a.m. - 4:30 p.m.
Weekends by appointment.

Admission - free

The museum, which opened February 9, 1985, recreates a neighborhood pharmacy of the 1930s. The museum committee, headed by pharmacist James Kuykendall, went about the task of gathering authentic equipment to re-create the 1930s pharmacy. More than 1,000 artifacts have been donated or purchased from areas in the southeast.

The collection includes a variety of crude drugs; medicines, liniments, lozenges, pills, and powders contained in glass bottles with cork stoppers; and a soda fountain to create an atmosphere of nostalgia of days gone by. The restoration includes a pressed tin ceiling, period light fixtures, and refinished oak flooring.

ARIZONA

Tucson

Adams Museum of Pharmacy and Medicine
10910 East Tanque Verde Road
Tucson, Arizona 85749
(520) 749-4538

Owned by Mrs. Ivor K. Adams.

Open by appointment only.

Admission - $2.00

An original nineteenth-century pharmacy, housed in its own building was saved from the wrecking ball in Chillecothe, Ohio, and reconstructed in Tucson, Arizona. The carved cherry fixtures contain the original glass-labeled stock bottles and contents, prescription and patent medicines with contents, tools of the trade, perfumes, and sundries. In one corner of the prescription compounding area is the doctor's walnut roll top desk over which are leather bound medical and pharmacy books. Across the room are examples of his instruments and medicines he used to treat the sick on his daily rounds. In addition to the usual items found in an apothecary of the nineteenth-century are collections of nursing bottles, poison bottles, bitters bottles, eye baths, boxes that contained various cures, medicine spoons, sick feeders, and unusual pharmaceutical memorabilia from around the world.

TUCSON

The History of Pharmacy Museum
University of Arizona College of Pharmacy
P.O. Box 210207, 1703 E. Mabel
Tucson, AZ 85721-0207
(520) 626-4065

Website http://www.pharmacy.arizona.edu/museum

Owned by the University of Arizona College of Pharmacy. Richard Wiedopf, curator.

Monday - Friday 8:00 a.m. - 5:00 p.m.

Admission - free

The museum was founded in 1966 and comprises three units. The History of Pharmacy Museum at the University of Arizona College of Pharmacy grew out of the work of Jesse Hurlbut, a former Tucson pharmacist and state pharmacy board inspector, who meticulously collected pharmacy items from around Arizona and elsewhere in the West. The museum opened in the old Pharmacy/Microbiology building on Main Campus and was moved to the current College of Pharmacy building at the Arizona Health Sciences Center in 1982.

The museum contains a collection of over 60,000 bottles, books, display cases, and scores of artifacts from Arizona (circa 1880 to 1930). Most impressive are several large drugstore fixtures form Arizona's territorial days; an impressive collection of 18 large show globes; hundreds of antique mortars and pestles; and over 65 feet of original display cases used in a Chicago pharmacy.

Through a self-guided tour, visitors can see a replica of a late nineteenth-century "botica" of the territorial Southwest, which contains original equipment and fixtures. A period pharmacy counter of the 1920s and '30s is furnished with various tools of the apothecary, supplies, and fixtures.

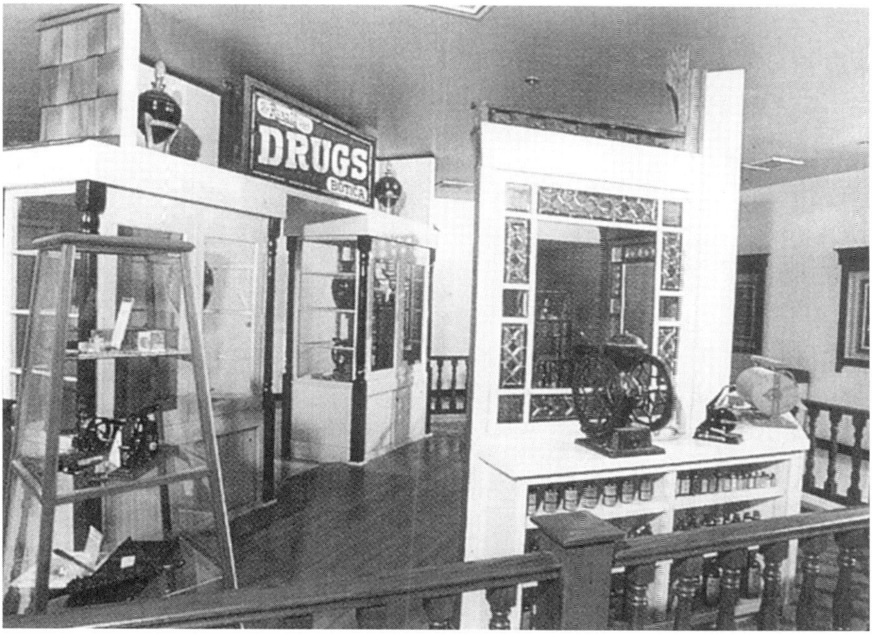

Drug store exhibit at the History of Pharmacy Museum
University of Arizona, Tucson, Arizona

PHOENIX

Medical Museum - Phoenix Baptist Hospital
6025 N. 20th Avenue
Phoenix, AZ 85015
(602) 249-0212

Daily 8:00 a.m. - 9:00 p.m.

Admission - free

An extensive display of pharmaceutical and medical antiques dating back to the American Revolution. Cases are in the main lobby and throughout the hospital's seven floors. On the same campus as Chris Ridge Nursing Home, there is a walk-in replica of a turn-of-the-century pharmacy and post office. There are additional displays in the new outpatient surgical center. The items are a loan from the collection of Robert E. Kravetz, M.D.

CALIFORNIA

BAKERSFIELD

Kern County Museum
3801 Chester Avenue
Bakersfield, CA 93301
(805) 861-2132

Owned and administered by County of Kern Board of Supervisors, State of California. Carola Rupert Enriquez, director.

Monday - Friday	8:00 a.m. - 5:00 p.m.
Saturday, Sunday, and holidays	10:00 a.m. - 5:00 p.m.

Admission - adults $5,00; senior citizens $4.00; children under 12, $3.00.

The original fixtures were built by Marion Carlock in 1890 and were donated by his daughter. The building originally housed the Carlock Feed & Grain Co. The exhibition was opened to the public in 1957 in this outdoor museum with displays and artifacts dating from about 1880 to 1945.

The apothecary shop furnishings include patent medicines (from Ayer's Sarsaparilla to Pinkham's Pink Pills), drug containers, show globes, and prescription files. Among over sixty other restorations is a physician's office and a dentist's office. The exhibits provide a nostalgic view of central California in its pioneering days.

BUENA PARK

Knott's Berry Farm
8039 Beach Boulevard
Buena Park, CA 90620
(714) 220-5200

Owned and operated by the Knott Family. Dana Hammontree, curator.

Summer	
Sunday - Thursday	9:00 a.m. - 11:00 p.m.
Friday and Saturday	9:00 a.m. - Midnight
Winter	
Monday - Friday	10:00 a.m. - 6:00 p.m.
Saturday	10:00 a.m. - 10:00 p.m.
Sunday	10:00 a.m. - 8:00 p.m.

Admission - adults $35.00; children under 12, $25.00

The original Ghost Town was developed in 1940 by Walter Knott (born 1889), intended as an integral part of the Berry Farm experience and adventure and to pay homage to the pioneering spirit and love for the "old west." Initially an 1868 gold-trail hotel contained a covered-wagon show. The buildings were dismantled from near Prescott, Arizona, and moved to Buena Park, California, where they were reinstalled on a 150-acre farm. Of special interest is an apothecary shop front in the Western Trail Museum. It exhibits a prescription department, stocks of medicinal bottles, tools, and artifacts of the apothecary art utilized in the "old west" from the 1860s to the end of the century; it is typical of California's mining communities of this era. Another important exhibit is the dental office of Dr. Lamuel Walker with period equipment and tools.

Columbia

Columbia State Historic Park
22708 Broadway
Columbia, CA 95310
(209) 532-0150

Managed by The California Parks and Recreation Department. Sherrin Grout, ranger.

Daily	9:30 a.m. - 4:30 p.m.

Admission - free

The pharmacy was presented to the State in 1957 by the California Pharmacists Association. It was licensed as a permanent display-only pharmacy museum of the gold-rush period by the Department of Professional and Vocational Standards. It depicts a California pharmacy of the late-nineteenth century with stock and fixtures. Another park exhibit on Main Street depicts a Chinese (medicinal) Herb Shop of the period 1852-1870.

Garden Grove

Pharmacy Restoration (Private)
12272 Lampson Ave.
Garden Grove, CA 92840
(714) 534-4467

Owned by L. & D. Serber. L. Serber M.D., director.

Open by appointment only.

Admission - free

This is a re-creation of an 1880s pharmacy with contents. Pharmacy artifacts on display include medical and surgical artifacts of the 1800s, antique medical furniture, and surgical sets.

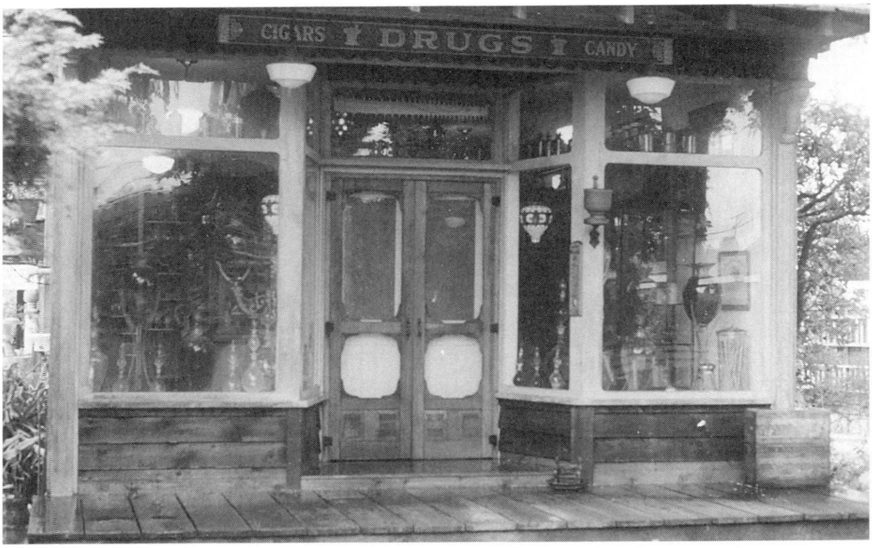

Exterior of 1880s pharmacy restoration.
Garden Grove, California

San Diego

Witfeld Old Town Drug Store
The Whaley House
2482 San Diego Avenue
San Diego, CA 92110
(619) 298-2482

Owned and operated by the Historical Shrine Foundation of San Diego County. June Reading, Director.

Spring/Summer
Tuesday - Sunday 10:00 a.m. - 4:00 p.m.
Fall/Winter
Wednesday - Sunday 10:00 a.m. - 4:00 p.m.

Admission - free

The Witfeld Old Town Drug Store Museum was inaugurated in 1969 under the direction of Mrs. James Reading in cooperation with the San Diego County and Southern California Pharmaceutical Associations. The restoration is named after the pharmaceutical-chemist Gustavus Witfeld, who was born near Cologne, Germany, on January 27, 1825. He became the city pharmacist of San Diego in 1868 and died there on September 15, 1894. The original building was restored on the Whaley House grounds and displays original furnishings; pharmaceutical implements; glass and ceramic containers; pill, suppository, and tablet machines; soap cutter; and percolators of the 1850s to the 1880s.

A physician's clinic with period equipment and tools is also attached to the pharmacy. Adjacent to the museum is a botanical garden with herbal spices reminiscent of a bygone era.

San Francisco

Museum of Ophthalmology
655 Beach Street
San Francisco, CA 94109-1336
(415) 561-8502

Operated by the Foundation of the American Academy of Ophthalmology. Licia Wells, director.

Open by appointment only.

Admission - free

Established in 1980 to increase interest in ophthalmology through the preservation and interpretation of its history. The museum displays an assortment of eyecups, pharmaceuticals, nostrums, and sundries (1830-1930).

STOCKTON

The Haggin Museum, Victory Park
1201 North Pershing
Stockton, CA 95203
(209) 462-1566

Managed by The Haggin Museum. Tod Ruhstaller, director.

Tuesday - Sunday 1:30 p.m. - 5:00 p.m.

Admission - free

This turn-of-the-century pharmacy restoration features materials once part of the E.S. Holden Drug Store in Stockton. In the same exhibition area is a late nineteenth- and early twentieth-century Chinese herb shop, also from the Stockton area.

STOCKTON

University of the Pacific School of Pharmacy
751 Brookside Road
Stockton, CA 95211
(209) 946-2561

E-mail proppen@uop.edu

Owned and operated by the University of the Pacific School of Pharmacy.

Open by appointment only - contact the Dean's Office.

Admission - free

The collection, a gift from pharmacist Carl D. Lovotti of San Francisco, California, consists of 55 majolica drug jars, plates, flasks, pitchers, and plaques from Castelli, Savona, Urbino, and Faenza dating from the fifteenth through the eighteenth centuries. The collection is displayed in mahogany showcases acquired from a nineteenth-century pharmacy in Fresno, California.

COLORADO

Fair Play

South Park City Museum
100 4th Street
P.O. Box 634
Fair Play, CO 80440
(719) 836-2387

Affiliated with South Park Historical Foundation, Inc. Carol A. Davis, general manager.

May 15 - October 15
Daily 9:00 a.m. - 5:00 p.m.

Admission - adults $5.00; senior citizens $4.00; children $2.00.

Founded in 1957, this historic village museum is on the site of a post-Civil War mining town of about 1879 with authentic buildings from the 1860s to 1880s. It includes temporary and permanent displays depicting lifestyles, trades, and professions of the period, including the J. A. Merriam Drug Store restoration.

Fort Garland

Fort Garland Museum
P. O. Box 368
Fort Garland, CO 81133
(303) 379-3512

Owned by the State Historical Society of Colorado, and operated by the Colorado History Museum, 1300 Broadway, Denver, CO 80203; (303) 866-3917. Rick Manzanares, director.

April - October
Daily 9:00 a.m. - 5:00 p.m.
November - March
Thursday - Monday 8:00 a.m. - 4:00 p.m.

Admission - adults $2.50; senior citizens $2.00; children (6-16) $1.50; children under 6 and members free.

This is a restoration of an historic fort once commanded by Kit Carson. The fort was active between 1858 and 1883. The exhibit includes one case containing a Civil War medical field kit as well as medicinal containers, surgical and medical instruments, and equipment representing the health professions in Colorado Territory during the Civil War period.

CONNECTICUT

HARTFORD

The Menczer Museum of Medicine and Dentistry
230 Scarborough Street
Hartford, CT 06105
(860) 236-5613

Owned and operated by the Hartford Medical Society and Hartford Dental Society. Bernard Kosto, M.D., and Adolph Bushell, D.D.S., curators.

Monday - Friday 9:00 a.m. - 4:30 p.m.
Weekends by appointment.

Admission - adults, $2.00 contribution

The museum displays instruments, equipment and furnishings, including pharmaceuticals dating from the nineteenth-century.

MYSTIC

Mystic Seaport - The Museum of America and the Sea
75 Greenmanville Avenue
P.O. Box 6000
Mystic, CT 06355-0990
(860) 572-0711

Website www.mysticseaport.org

Owned by Mystic Seaport Museum, Inc. J. Revell Carr, Director.

Call for hours.

Admission - adults $16.00; youth (6 - 12) $8.00; children under 5 and U.S. military service personnel in uniform admitted free.

Mystic Seaport is an outdoor maritime museum that tells the stories of America and the sea. Installed in 1964, the Bringhurst Apothecary Shop was rearranged in 1975 to represent more accurately the 1870-1885 period. The restoration centers around the century-old original fixtures of the pharmacy pharmacist Joseph Bringhurst (1767-1834) and his son Ferris (1807-1880). The father moved from Philadelphia, Pennsylvania, to Wilmington, Delaware, in 1793 where he established a pharmacy. The fixtures were fitted with period pharmaceutical equipment and artifacts (1870s to 1900).

Displayed are fine examples of show globes, medicine bottles and jars, mortars and pestles, weights and scales, leech jars, ear trumpet, glycerin dispenser, spices, dye cabinet and paint pigments, pill tiles, powder folders, tincture presses, patent medicines, kerosene-oil dispenser, and medicine chests as well as material to refurbish ships' medicine chests.

New Canaan

The Monroe-Cody Drug Store
13 Oenoke Ridge
New Canaan, CT 06840
(203) 966-1776

Owned by the New Canaan Historical Society.

Tuesday - Saturday 9:30 a.m. - 4:30 p.m.

Admission - free

When Main Street was widened during the late summer of 1965, this town landmark was donated by the son and daughters of pharmacist James J. Cody to the Historical Society. The original pharmacy was established in 1845 by Samuel Cook Silliman. In 1854, the pharmacy was sold to Lucius M. Monroe who installed the present fixtures and renovated the shop. It was known then as the New Canaan Drug Store. In 1918, pharmacist Cody, who had been long associated with Monroe, bought it and directed the business until his death. Here at the annex of the Town House, the elegant interior fixtures, apothecary tools, patent medicines, and advertising signs are displayed, portraying a representative image of the pre-Civil War American pharmacy.

New Haven

Cushing/Whitney Medical Library
Yale University
P.O. Box 208014
333 Cedar Street
New Haven, CT 06510
(203) 785-4354

Website www.med.yale.edu/library/historical

Owned and operated by the Cushing/Whitney Medical Library, Yale University. Toby A. Appel, Historical Librarian.

Monday - Friday 9:00 a.m. - 4:30 p.m.

Admission - free

The contents of the pharmacy collection were a gift of Dr. Edward Clark Streeter (1874-1947). They include American items (1845-1880, eastern Connecticut), including a tall herb cabinet dated 1880. Hand-blown American glassware and pill machines are from Mystic and Hope Valley. European faience and glassware, mortars, and drug jars dated 1500-1800. Also of pharmaceutical interest is the remarkable Streeter collection of weights, balances, gold coin scales, and linear and bulk measures from the ancient civilization to those of nineteenth-century Europe and America.

The exhibition is housed in the Yale Medical School entrance foyer and in the Yale Medical Library. The library also houses medical and surgical instruments, kits, saddle bags, medals, bookplates, prints, drawings, and portraits. Other artifacts include obstetrical forceps, scarificators, eyeglasses, microscopes, endoscopes, catheters, probes, vaporizers, and atomizers.

STORRS

The University of Connecticut School of Pharmacy
372 Fairfield Road
Storrs, CT 06269-2092
(860) 486-2129

E-mail gerald@uconnvm.uconn.edu

Owned and operated by the University of Connecticut School of Pharmacy. Michael Gerald, dean.

Open weekdays during school hours.

Admission - free

Donated in 1967 by Edith Smith Mogull in memory of her late husband, pharmacist Edward Mogull, the collection includes drug jars, mortars and pestles, glass bottles, show globes, medico-pharmaceutical books, and other related pharmaceutical antiques. The collection is displayed in the hallways of the Pharmacy Research Institute building at the University of Connecticut School of Pharmacy.

PILL SPATULAS.

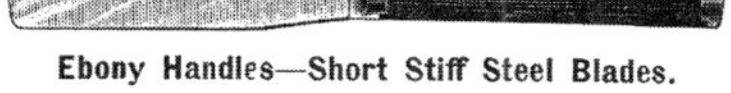

Ebony Handles—Short Stiff Steel Blades.

	Per doz.
$2\frac{1}{2}$ inch blade	$7 00
$3\frac{1}{2}$ inch blade	7 75

DISTRICT OF COLUMBIA

WASHINGTON, D.C.

The National Museum of Health and Medicine
Walter Reed Army Medical Center
Georgia Avenue and Elder Street, NW
Washington, D.C. 20306-6000
(202) 782-2200

Governed by the Armed Forces Institute of Pathology. Adrianne Noe, director.

Daily 10:30 a.m.- 5:30 p.m.

Admission - contribution

The National Museum of Health and Medicine was founded as the Army Museum by the United States Surgeon General of the Army, William A. Hammond, in 1862. From 1887 to 1969, it shared a red-brick building on the Mall next to the Smithsonian at Seventh Street and Independence Avenue, S.W., with the Army Medical Library (later the Armed Forces Medical Library and presently the National Library of Medicine), as conceived in the visionary plans of Dr. John Shaw Billings (director, 1865-1895). When the building was demolished, the museum collections were moved to their present quarters. The exhibits were reopened to the public on May 2, 1971. The exhibition displays pathological specimens, military and medical artifacts, and instruments, many of which predate the Civil War. The museum is especially noted for its historical microscope collection.

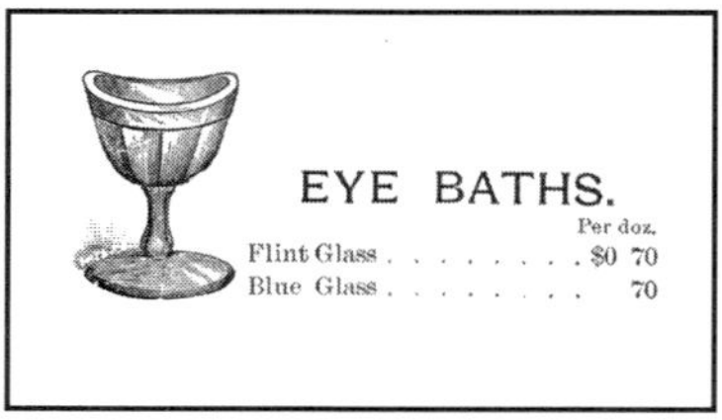

Supplement to:
Pharmacy Museums and Historical Collections in the United States and Canada

by George Griffenhagen and Ernst W. Stieb

ARIZONA

Medical Museum
Phoenix Baptist Hospital Lobby
6025 N. 20th Avenue
Phoenix, AZ 85015
(602) 249-0212
Open 8 a.m.-9 p.m. daily. Free admission.
Medical and pharmaceutical antiques dating to the American Revolutionary period. Items on display loaned to the hospital by Robert Kravetz, M.D.

GEORGIA

Georgia Agrirama
State Museum of Agriculture
I-75 and 8th St., P.O. Box Q
Tifton, GA 31793
(912) 386-3344
Wilbur N. Willis, Executive Director. Open Mon.-Sat. 9:30 a.m.-5:30 p.m.
A living history museum depicting rural life of a century ago. Includes a 19th-century drugstore with working soda fountain where beverages are served.

ILLINOIS

Blackberry Historical Farm Village
R.R. 3 Box 591 Galena Blvd. & Barnes Rd.
Aurora, IL 60506
(708) 892-5664
Sue Topp, Museum Registrar. Open seasonally: daily May-Labor Day, then Fri.-Sun. only through mid-Oct. Hours 10 a.m.-4:30 p.m. Admission charged.
"Early Streets of Aurora" museum features storefronts and turn-of-the-century merchandise including an Apothecary Shop. Over 2000 pharmaceutical objects in the collection.

Museum of Science and Industry
Walgreen Drug Store, Chicago 1901
5700 S. Lake Shore Dr.
Chicago, IL 60637
(312) 940-3033/3034
The new exhibit is a faithful reproduction of the first Walgreen Store on the main floor in "Yesterday's Main Street" section of the museum. (Update to monograph in *Pharmacy Museums*, 1988, p. 19.)

Health Education Center Exhibition
The Robert Crown Center for Health Education
21 Salt Creek Lane
Hinsdale, IL 60521
(312) 325-1900
Dr. John P. Zaremba, Executive Director. Open 9-3 Mon.-Fri. mid-Sept.-mid-June for school groups only; 3-4:30 p.m. Mon.-Fri. for other than school groups; and 9-2 Mon.-Fri. mid-June-mid-Sept.
Various health education displays including assorted collections of medications, drug containers, and tools; lectures and films related to drug abuse are given periodically.

MICHIGAN

Greenfield Village & Henry Ford Museum
Oakwood Blvd.,
Dearborn, MI 48121
(313) 271-1620
Owned and operated by Edison Institute, Inc., Dorothy Tasker, Marketing Manager. Hours 9-5 daily year around except Thanksgiving, Christmas and New Year's Day. \$10.50 adults; \$5.25 children; \$9.50 senior citizens.
Pharmaceutical utensils, tools, drug jars, glassware, etc., not currently on display.

NEW JERSEY

Old Village in the Historic Towne of Smithville
Route 9
Absecon (town of Smithville) NJ 08201
(609) 652-7777
Owned and operated by the Historic Smithville Inns, Inc., a subsidiary of ABC, Inc., Catherine T. Hilferty, Marketing Administrator. Hours 10-3 Tues.-Fri. June; 10-5 Tues.-Fri. July-Aug.; 11:30-5 Sat.-Sun. Sept.-Oct.
Adults \$2.50; students \$1.50; under 5 free; special rates for senior citizens.
Part of the historical village is a restored 19th-century drugstore.

OHIO

History of the Health Sciences Library and Museum
University of Cincinnati Medical Center
Cincinnati, OH 45267
(513) 872-5120
Billie Broaddus, Director. Open Mon.-Fri.
Rare and old books and journals, manuscripts, medical archives, hospital records, medical instruments, photographs, memorabilia, and ceramics.

Edward B. Ayres Drug Store
114 E. Main Street
Hillsboro, OH 45133
(513) 393-1629
Owned and operated by the Hillcrest Pharmacy, Inc., John Fuller, Pharmacist/Manager. Open 9-6 Mon., Tues., Thurs., Sat.; 1-6 Wed. Authentic fixtures in 1808 building with many old medicines and artifacts.

PENNSYLVANIA

Museum and Pharmaceutical Exhibits
The Philadelphia College of Pharmacy and Science
43rd Street and Kingsessing Avenue
Philadelphia, PA 19104
(215) 386-5800
Ara der Marderosian, Curator. Open weekdays during school hours; free. Exhibits at the first pharmacy school in the U.S. include a general pharmacy museum, the George Glenworth Pharmacy shop (opened in 1812), the Bohlander Drugstore, and the Joseph England Library collections.

SOUTH CAROLINA

Aiken County Historical Museum
433 Newberry St., S.W.
Aiken, SC 29801
(803) 642-2015
Owned and operated by Aiken County Historical Commission. Nana Farris, Director. Open 9:30-4:30 Tues.-Fri.; 2-5 p.m. 1st Sun. of each month. The Henry Moody Drug Store exhibit inlcudes the fixtures and inventory that were in it when it closed in 1951, featuring a 19th-century soda fountain.

SOUTH DAKOTA

Humphrey Drug
233 Dakota St.
Huron, SD 57350
(605) 352-4064
Owned and operated by Ralph and Bonnie Gosch. Open Mon.-Sat. 9-5.
Hubert H. Humphrey's family drugstore, started by his father in 1903.

Wall Drug Apothecary Shoppe & Pharmacy Museum
510 Main Street
Wall, SD 57790
(605)279-2175
Owned and operated by Bill Hustead. Open 6:30 a.m.-9:30 p.m. summer months; closed Nov. 15-April.
Fashioned after the original drug store which was located across the street from the present location and founded in 1931. Over 400 pharmacutical artifacts.

VERMONT

The Apothecary Shop
Shelburne Museum
U.S. Route 7
Shelburne, VT 05482
(802) 985-3344
Brian Alexander, Director. Open 9-5 daily mid-May to mid-Oct. Adults $12; children $4.50; under 6 free.
Pharmacy reconstruction with authentic fixtures and shelf ware.

ONTARIO, CANADA

History of Contraception Museum
19 Green Belt Drive
Don Mills, Ontario M3C 1L9 Canada
(416) 449-9444
Heather Bennett, Director. Open by appointment only to medical professionals.
Methods of contraception from 1550 B.C. to the future.

Washington, D.C.

National Museum of American History
Pharmacy Collections
Division of Science, Medicine and Society
Smithsonian Institution
14th and Constitution Avenue, N.W.
Washington, D.C. 20560
(202) 357-2145

Governed by the Smithsonian Institution, Spencer Crew, director; Ramunas Kondratas, curator/acting assistant director for history.

Daily 10:00 a.m. - 5:30 p.m.
Collection open to researchers by appointment only.

Admission - free

The pharmacy collections at the National Museum of American History are the largest and most comprehensive of their kind in the United States. They date back to the crude drug specimens displayed at the 1876 Centennial exhibition in Philadelphia and then transferred to the United States National Museum, where in 1881 they became a part of a new Section of Materia Medica, which is now the Division of Science, Medicine and Society. They document the history of pharmacy and pharmaceutical manufacturing in the United States from the eighteenth to the twentieth centuries and are rich in objects and supporting documentation in every major collecting category—products, containers, tools, laboratory and manufacturing equipment, prescription and manufacturing records, furnishings, photographs, advertising materials, and trade literature. The 1,100 piece Bristol-Myers Squibb collection consists of European pharmaceutical artifacts from the fifteenth through the nineteenth centuries.

The Hall of Medical Sciences, which contained the pharmaceutical history displays, closed in 1991 to make way for the *Science in American Life* exhibit and the Hands-On Science Center. The next major exhibit, tentatively titled *Health in America,* should premiere at the turn of the millennium.

For an overview and history of the pharmacy collection, please see the article "The Pharmacy Collections" by D. L. Weudt and E.W. Jentsch in *Caduceus: A Museum Journal; for Medicine and the Health Sciences* 13, no. 3 (1997): 33-42. This entire issue of the journal is devoted to the topic "150 Years of Collecting Medical History at the Smithsonian Institution."

FLORIDA

Ft. Lauderdale

Health Museum Nova Southeastern University
Health Professions Division
3200 South University Drive
Ft. Lauderdale, FL 33328
(954) 262 1300

Owned and operated by Nova Southeastern University. Paul Magalian, director.

Monday - Friday	8:00 a.m. - 5:00 p.m.

Admission - free

The museum is located in the main entrance of the Health Professions Division of the University. The museum has an extensive collection of pharmaceutical glassware, show globes, jars, mortars and pestles, scales, books, suppository molds and presses, prescription files, and pill tiles. Seven display cases are devoted to pharmaceutical equipment and artifacts of historical and professional interest.

Miami Springs

Miami Springs Pharmacy and Museum
45 Curtiss Parkway
Miami Springs, FL 33166
(305) 888-5250

Owned and operated by John Stadnik.

Sunday - Friday	9:00 a.m. - 6:00 p.m.
Saturday	10:00 a.m. - 4:00 p.m.

Admission - free

The museum is located on the ground floor of the Clune Building (1925) built by Glenn H. Curtiss of aviation fame. The Miami Springs Pharmacy opened in 1946 in this historic site. The museum features hundreds of jars, bottles, chemicals, herbs, oils and ointments. A complete Rexall collection includes 30 gallon bottles of tonics, tinctures, fluid extracts, which were re-bottled for prescription use. Two typewriters, 12 pharmacy scales and balances, and over 40 mortars and pestles are on display. A wall of pharmaceutical text books are featured with prescription files and narcotic registers. Historic portraits, photographs, pharmacy awards and certificates, and all the usual items needed for compounding and dispensing are also displayed.

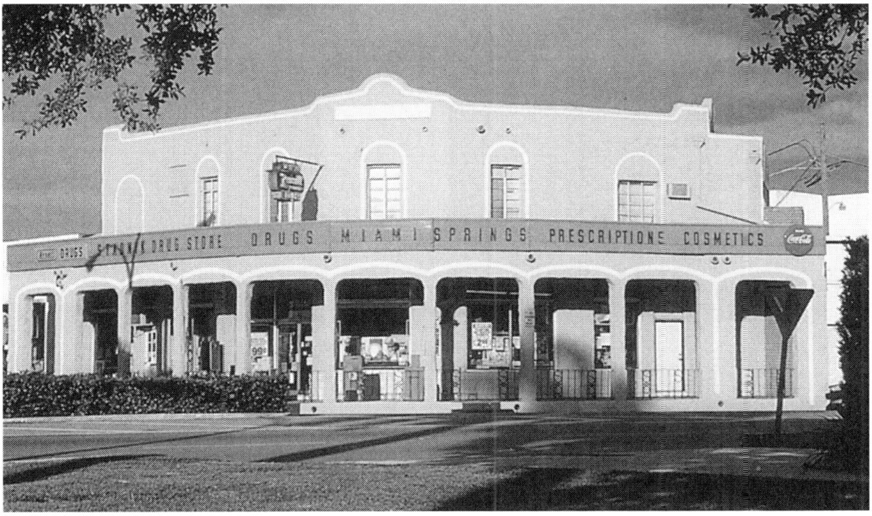

Miami Springs Pharmacy and Museum. The Clune Building also houses the Miami Springs Historical Musuem. Miami Springs, Florida.

PENSACOLA

Pensacola Historical Museum
115 E. Zaragosa Street
Pensacola, FL 32501
(850) 433-1559

Owned and operated by Pensacola Historical Society. Sandra Johnson, assistant curator.

Museum
Monday - Saturday 9:00 a.m. - 4:30 p.m.
Library
Tuesday-Thursday and Saturday 10:00 a.m. - 3:00 p.m.

Admission - Museum $1.00; Library $2.00.

The museum features the history of Pensacola and northwest Florida from pre-historic Indians to the present. The pharmacy display includes bottles from local pharmacies and assorted medical and pharmaceutical artifacts.

GEORGIA

ATHENS

University of Georgia College of Pharmacy
D.W. Brooks Drive at Green Street
Athens, GA 30602
(404) 542-1911

Owned and operated by the University of Georgia College of Pharmacy.

Open by appointment during school hours - contact the Dean's Office.

Admission - free

Eight panels display pharmaceutical artifacts of historical and professional interest. The exhibits rotate periodically. One of the more unique artifacts on permanent display is the mortar and pestle used by Dr. Crawford W. Long, the first person to use diethyl ether for surgical anesthesia. Dr. Long and his brother Robert opened a pharmacy on Broad Street in Athens, Georgia. It was here that Crawford and Robert Long practiced both medicine and pharmacy.

ATLANTA

Southern School of Pharmacy
Mercer University
3001 Mercer University Drive
Atlanta, GA 30341
(770) 986-3282

Owned and operated by Mercer University. Trudy Kelly, archivist, Swilly Library.

Open by appointment only - contact the Dean's Office.

Admission - free

The lobby features two exhibit cases with fixtures from an Atlanta pharmacy of the early 1900s. Displayed are tools of the apothecary, including jars, proprietary medicines, an iron mortar and pestle of the Revolutionary period, old prescriptions, apothecary chest (c. 1800), typewriter with pharmaceutical symbols, and pill roller. Framed composite photographs of graduating classes are displayed in the hallway. The Swilley Library Archives contains the archives of the Southern School of Pharmacy (1903-1959), archives of the Mercer University Southern School of Pharmacy (1959-present), yearbooks, catalogs, publications, photographs, framed diplomas, and pharmaceutical artifacts. The Swilley Library Special Collections rooms house nineteenth- century editions of dispensatories, APhA publications, and other assorted pharmacy related materials.

COLUMBUS

The Pemberton House and Apothecary
11 Seventh Street
Columbus, GA 31901
(706) 322-0756

Owned and operated by the Historic Columbus Foundation, Inc. Mrs. R. Chris Peebles, executive director.

Tours

Monday - Friday	11:00 a.m. and 3:00 p.m.
Weekends	2:00 p.m.

Admission - $3.00 for guide fee.

The Pemberton House and Apothecary was moved to its present location from its 1855 site and was restored to its original decor as a four-room Victorian cottage that was occupied by Dr. John Stith Pemberton (1833-1888), a Georgia pharmacist. The kitchen has been furnished to resemble a "chemical laboratory" of the nineteenth century. It was in Columbus that Dr. Pemberton began preparing and dispensing his "cool, cordial and refreshing drinks" for his customers and regularly advertised them in the *Columbus Enquirer-Sun*. These "concoctions" and "draughts" often included one called "French Wine of Cocoa— ideal nerve tonic and stimulant," that was the forerunner of Coca-Cola.

Dr. Pemberton and his family moved from Columbus to Atlanta where in 1887 he sold the secret of the Coca-Cola formula for $1,750 to pharmacist Asa G. Candler, founder of the Coca-Cola Company. Dr. Pemberton died in Atlanta in 1888.

On display are period fixtures, including a Charles Tuft soda fountain. Other tools in the exhibit include a pill tile; spatulas for mixing ointments and salves; mortars and pestles; perfume; and Coca-Cola bottles. Recently acquired is the extensive Dr. Jesse L. Miller antique Coca-Cola Memorabilia Collection.

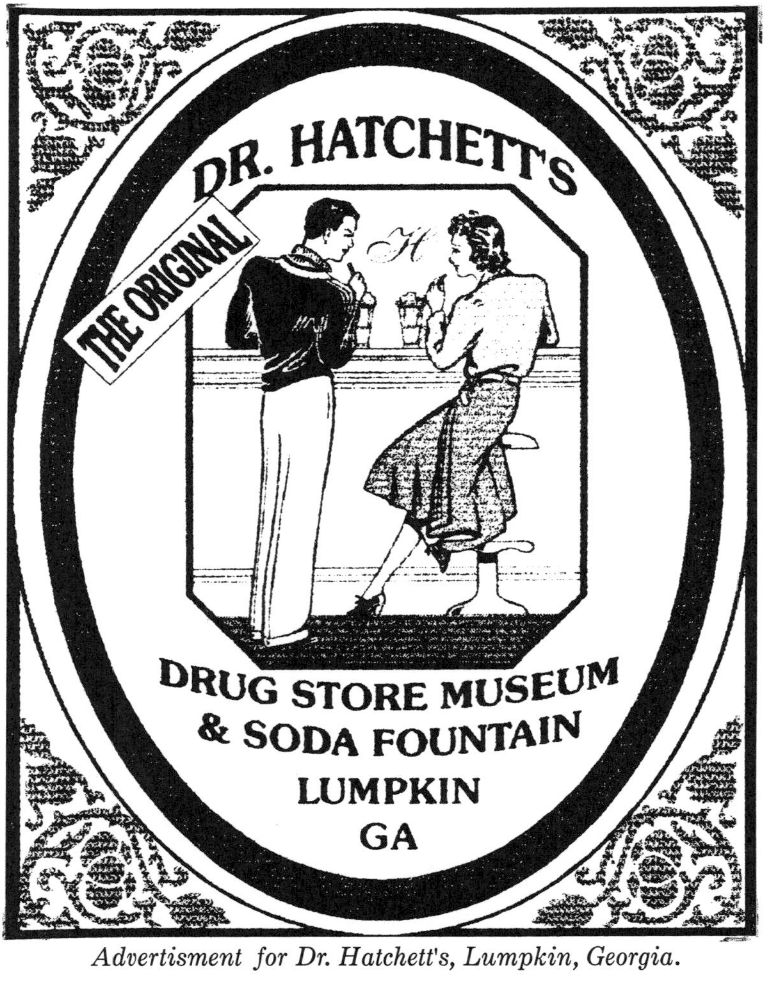

Advertisment for Dr. Hatchett's, Lumpkin, Georgia.

Lumpkin

Dr. Hatchett's Drug Store Museum
Main Street on the Square
Box 1056
Lumpkin, GA 31815
(912) 838-6924

E-mail AMoyeIII@Prodigy.net

Operated by Stewart County Historical Commission.
Andy Moye, curator.

Saturday, Tuesday-Thursday	11:00 a.m. - 5:00 p.m.
Friday	11:00 a.m. - 7:30 p.m.
Sunday	12:00 p.m. - 5:00 p.m.

Admission- free

This drugstore includes both pharmacy and medical items dating back to the Civil War. Most of the collection is from the early twentieth-century but the original founder was a Civil War physician. The result is an unusually broad collection of apothecary jars, patent medicines, pharmaceutical and medical equipment, cabinets and displays, as well as general merchandise.

Lumpkin

Westville Historic Handicrafts
P. O. Box 1850
Lumpkin, GA 31815
(912) 838-6310

Owned and operated by the Westville Historic Handicrafts, Inc.
Matthew Moye, curator.

Tuesday - Saturday	10:00 a.m. - 5:00 p.m.
Sunday	1:00 p.m. - 5:00 p.m.

Admission - adults $8.00; senior citizens, military, and college students $7.00; students grades K-12 $4.00.

Westville Historic Handicrafts is a restored village of thirty-five buildings and shops. Featured is a restoration of the office and apothecary shop of Dr. William L. Paullin established in 1845 in Fort Gaines, Georgia. It contains original period furnishings including medical equipment, medicine kits and tools, dental instruments, herbal charts, desks, and a collection of mortars and pestles.

ILLINOIS

AURORA

Blackberry Historical Farm Village
100 S. Barnes Road
Aurora, IL 60506
(630) 892-5664

E-mail dheffernan@iyc.hpc.org

Operated by the Fox Valley Park District. Lorraine Beasley, registrar.

May-Labor Day
Daily 10:00 a.m. - 4:30 p.m.
Labor Day - mid-October
Friday - Sunday 10:00 a.m. - 4:30 p.m.

Admission - adults $7.00; senior citizens $6.00; children 2-12 $6.00.

The"Early Street of Aurora" museum features storefronts and turn-of-the-century merchandise including an apothecary shop. Over 2000 pharmaceutical objects are in the collection, and the contents of an original turn-of-the-century pharmacy.

No. 40

GRADUATED MEDICINE SPOON.

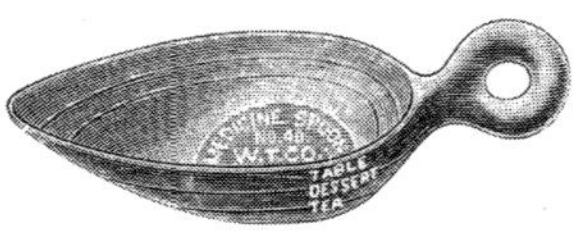

GLASS.

To Measure Tea, Dessert and Tablespoonfuls.

No. 40 . . . . $13 00 per gross.

Furnished also with lettering in Spanish.

Two Gross in Original Package.

This Spoon can be furnished in lots of two gross and upward with customer's name, etc., pressed in the glass as an advertisement. The lettering is pressed on the bottom of the spoon, so as to be read from above, but without affecting the smoothness of the bowl inside.

CHICAGO

International Museum of Surgical Science
1524 North Lake Shore Drive
Chicago, IL 60610
(312) 642-6502 ext. 315

Website www.imss.org

Owned and operated by the International College of Surgeons.
Margaret Schlesinger, curator.

Tuesday - Saturday	10:00 a.m. - 4:00 p.m.
Sunday	11:00 a.m. - 5:00 p.m.

Admission - $3.00 suggested donation.

Among thirty-two rooms and halls displaying artifacts, models, instruments, illustrations of the history of surgery and therapy, and the story of mankind's continuing struggle against suffering and disease, is a reconstructed late nineteenth-century pharmacy. Many of its fixtures and pieces of equipment date back to the last quarter of the nineteenth century. These were furnishings and artifacts preserved from an 1873 pharmacy owned by Charles W. Sackett (d. 1917) and Fred C. Taber (d. 1880) of Addison, New York. Additional fixtures, equipment, and merchandise came from the apothecary shop of Dr. Uriah C. Jones (ca. 1882) of Breda, Iowa.

In this exhibit are two prescription counters, display cases, period lighting fixtures and shelf ware, and drawers labeled with the names of stored herbs. Also on display are show globes, scales and weights, patent medicines, pharmacy records, registration certificates, and a mannequin of a practicing pharmacist. The exhibit was inaugurated on November 30, 1966, under the auspices of Charles R. Walgreen, Jr.

CHICAGO

Museum of Science and Industry
57th Street and South Lake Shore Drive
Chicago, IL 60637
(773) 684-1414

Website www.msichicago.org

Owned and operated by the Museum of Science and Industry. Michael Sarna, curator.

Memorial Day - Labor Day	
Daily	9:30 a.m. - 5:30 p.m.
Balance of year	
Monday - Friday	9:30 a.m. - 4:00 p.m.
Saturday, Sunday, and Holidays	9:30 a.m. - 5:30 p.m.

Admission- Museum: adults $6.00, senior citizens $5.00; children 3-11 $2.50; children under 3 free.

Occupying the reconstructed Fine Arts Building of the 1893 Columbia Exposition, the museum opened in 1933. Oriented toward advances in pure and applied sciences and industrial technology, it displays several exhibits on health and biology; a giant 16-foot walk-through human heart, hatching of live baby chicks, and full-size transparent mannequin of a woman to show bodily function.

Most relevant, however, is the old pharmacy exhibition, in Yesterday's Main Street, a nostalgic recreation of the original Walgreen's Drug Company opened by Charles R. Walgreen, Sr., in 1901. Fixtures and pharmacy tools span the late nineteenth through early twentieth centuries and include patent medicines, herbal remedies, cosmetics, tobacco products, soap, trusses, drug jars, and prescription books. The original Walgreen's Drug Company was located at 4134 S. Cottage Grove Avenue, Northwest of the museum.

HINSDALE

Health Education Center Exhibition
The Robert Crown Center for Health Education
21 Salt Creel Lane
Hinsdale, IL 60521
(630) 325-1900

E-mail rcche@anet-chi.com

Governed by Board of Directors. John P. Zarema, executive director.

Mid September - mid June
Daily 3:00 p.m. - 4:30 p.m.

Admission - adults - 3rd grade $3.00; 2nd grade - preschool $2.75.

Various health education displays are included in these assorted collections of medications, drug containers and tools. Lectures and films related to drug abuse are given daily.

INDIANA

EVANSVILLE

Evansville Museum of Arts and Science
411 S.E. Riverside Drive
Evansville, IN 47713
(812) 425-2406

Owned and operated by the Evansville Museum of Arts and Science. John W. Streetman III, director.

Tuesday - Saturday 10:00 a.m. - 5:00 p.m.
Sunday 12:00 p.m.- 5:00 p.m.

Admission - free

The museum includes a restoration of the office and apothecary shop of Dr. William Morton Elliott, who was a graduate of the Evansville Medical College in 1853. The exhibit was named in honor of Hugh McGary, who in 1812 purchased 200 acres that later became the site of the incorporated town of Evansville.

The exhibit includes drug jars, medicine bottles, show globes, microscopes, nursing bottles, and tools of the apothecary, including pill tiles and machines, konseals, a cork press, measures, mortars and pestles, scales, drug mills, and suppository molds. It also contains medical and surgical equipment, including scarificators, syringes, lancets, an amputation kit, splints, and obstetric tools, as well as Dr. Elliott's medical diploma, textbooks, class cards, his thesis, and a letter of recommendation signed by members of the faculty of the Evansville Medical College.

Evansville

Bristol-Myers
2404 West Pennsylvania Street
Evansville, IN 47721
(812) 429-5000

Owned and operated by Mead Johnson Nutritionals, a division of Bristol-Myers Squibb Company. P. J. Paradossi, associate director of public affairs.

Monday - Friday 7:30 a.m. - 4:00 p.m.

Admission - free

A large exhibit case of pediatric antiques is displayed in the lobby of the administration building. The company was started in Jersey City, New Jersey, in 1905 by Edward Mead Johnson. The company moved to Evansville in 1915 and merged with Bristol-Myers Company in 1967. It was a chemical manufacturing plant, then turned to medical and sterile surgical supplies, and eventually became a leader in the field of infant nutrition. Mead Johnson developed an interest in collecting pediatric and pharmaceutical objects related to child health and nutritional products, which are represented in the display.

Indianapolis

Hook's American Drug Store Museum
Indiana State Fairgrounds
1180 East 38th Street
Indianapolis, IN 46205
(317) 924-5886

E-mail HookAmeRx@aol.com

Operated by Hook's American Drug Store Museum, Inc. James M. Rogers, executive director.

Tuesday - Sunday 11:00 a.m. - 4:00 p.m.

Admission - $2.00 donation suggested.

Since 1966, Hook's American Drug Store & Pharmacy Museum has brought its millions of visitors into sharp focus with a historical slice of hometown, America's most important health and social center: The American Drug Store. Its ornate set of ash, walnut, oak, and maple furnishings were in use from 1849 to 1962 in the small Indiana town of Cambridge City on the Old National Road.

In addition to the broad collection of drugstore and pharmacy artifacts, a vintage 1880s soda fountain regularly offers ice cream sodas, phosphates, fountain Cokes, and other treats to delight its visitors. Candy, novelties and many souvenir items and collectibles are available for sale.

In 1994, the Hook's Museum was donated to the private Hook Drug Foundation, Inc. by Revco (now CVS). Revco had acquired the rich asset when purchasing the remnants of the Indiana-based Hook's Drug Chain (1900-1985), from the original founder/owner. The Hook's Museum, which is perhaps the largest of its kind, today, is being developed into a national drugstore and pharmacy museum to reflect on pharmacy's past, present and future. A new museum will be established in two historic buildings located in downtown Indianapolis. A working Soda Fountain Emporium and Museum plus a 1950s Drugstore/Museum Gift Shop will open for business in early 2000. On October 5, 2000, the 100th Anniversary of the Founding of the Hook Drug Company, the museum and education center will be dedicated.

MITCHELL

Spring Mill State Park
State 60 E
P.O. Box 376
Mitchell, IN 47446
(812) 849-4129

E-mail spring@tima.com

Owned and operated by the Department of Natural Resources.
Dave Williams, park historian.

April - October
Daily 8:30 a.m. - 4:30 p.m.

Admission - free

The restored pioneer village consists of 18 structures, including an operating grist mill (museum), general store/post office, apothecary, loom house, residences. etc., complete with fixtures, tools, and equipment of the pre-Civil period.

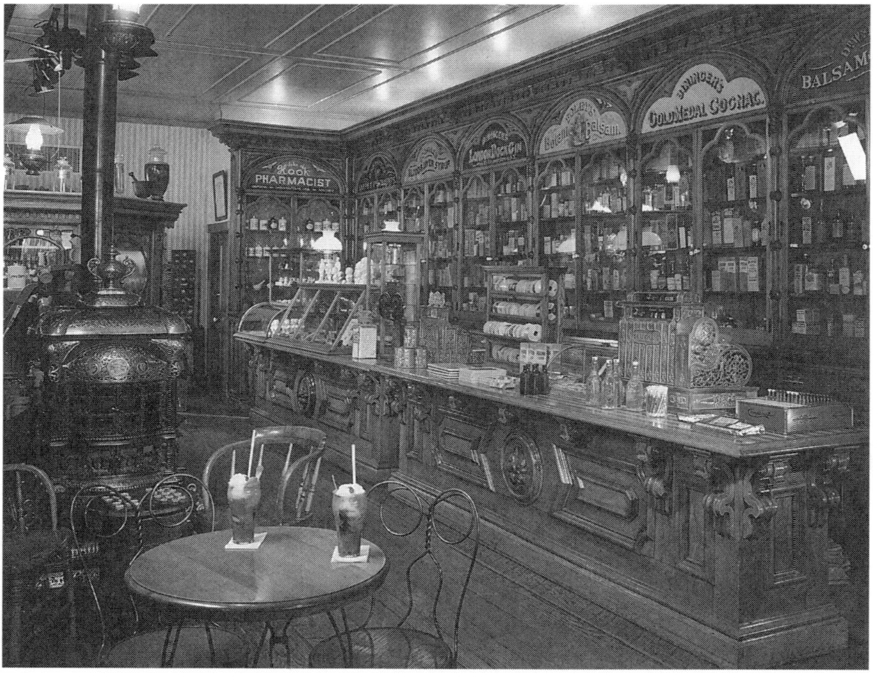

Interior Hook's American Drugstore Museum
Indianapolis, Indiana

IOWA

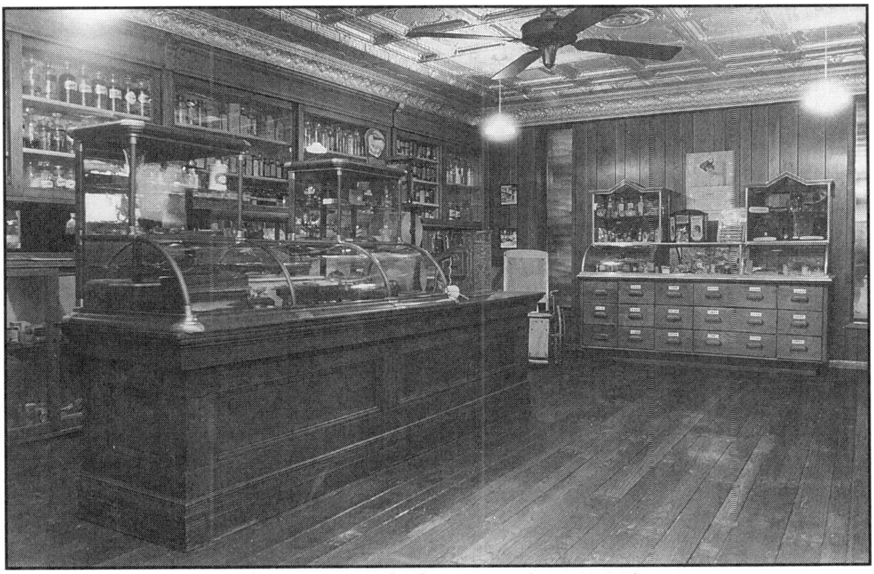

Reconstructed pharmacy (ca. 1906)
Druggists Mutual Insurance Company, Algona, Iowa.

ALGONA

Druggists Mutual Companies
808 Highway 18 West
Algona, IA 50511
(515) 295-2461

E-mail phmic.com

Owned and operated by the Pharmacists Mutual Foundation, Inc.
Shelly Brown, curator.

Monday - Friday 8:00 a.m. - 4:30 p.m.
Also by special appointment.

Admission - free

The reconstructed pharmacy, opened to the public in 1972, was patterned after a period-type pharmacy at the turn of the century when the Druggists Mutual Insurance Company was founded (1909). Among objects and sundries are glass-labeled shelf bottles, proprietary remedies, scales, perfumes, baby supplies, as well as various tools of the apothecary. This exhibit dramatizes the fact that this insurance company was organized and established by pharmacists and is still maintained exclusively by and for pharmacists and other health professionals.

CHARLES CITY

Floyd County Historical Society Museum
500 Gilbert Street
Charles City, IA 50616
(515) 228-1099

E-mail fchs@fia.net

Owned and operated by the Floyd County Historical Society.
Frank McKinney, director.

Monday - Friday	9:00 a.m. - 4:30 p.m.
May 1 - Labor Day	
Saturday	1:00 p.m. - 4:00 p.m.

Admission - adults $2.00; children 12-18 $1.00.

Many of the exhibits of the Floyd County Historical Society Museum include a drug and grocery business that started in 1873. The business was purchased in 1884 by John G. Legel and it remained in the family until 1961 when the building, the original furnishings, and the entire collection of pharmaceuticals were donated to the Society by John G. Legel, Jr.; the museum opened in 1962. Besides the soda fountain and the prescription counter, the shelves of this pharmacy are filled with drug bottles and jars, patent medicines, and scales, in addition to apothecary equipment, barrels and boxes of dry goods, household health supplies, remedies, and big glass jars of penny candy.

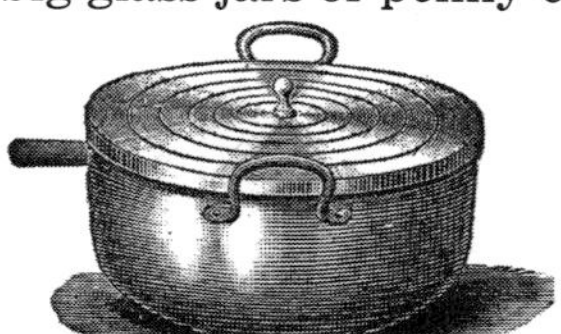

WATER BATHS.

Polished copper, tin-lined, with concentric copper rings, cover and steam escape.

Diameter.	Each.	Diameter.	Each.
4 inches, 3 rings . . .	$1 50	6 inches, 5 rings . . .	$2 50
5 inches, 4 rings . . .	2 00	8 inches, 6 rings . . .	4 00
5½ inches, 5 rings . . .	2 35	10 inches, 7 rings . . .	8 50

DISTILLING APPARATUS.

URBANDALE

Schafer Drugstore
Living History Farms
2600 N.W. 11th Street
Urbandale, IA 50322-3792
(515) 278-5286

Website www.lhf.org

Governed by Board of Directors. Steve Green, director.

Open May 1 - third Sunday in October

Admission - adults $8.00; senior citizens $7.00; children (4-12) $4.00.

The Schafer Drugstore is a replica of an 1875 small town Iowa drugstore. Contents include a prescription counter, display cases, retail counters, and laboratory case. Artifacts include apothecary jars, bottles, and compounding tools. Authentic and reproduction merchandise are also on display.

KANSAS

TOPEKA

Potwin Drugstore
Historic Ward Meade Park
124 N.W. Fillmore
Topeka, KS 66606
(785) 368-3888

Owned by the City of Topeka. Anita Wolgast, curator.

March - December

Tuesday - Saturday	10:00 a.m. - 4:00 p.m.
Sunday	12:00 p.m . - 4:00 p.m.

Admission - free to drugstore (other parts of park require a nominal charge).

Opened in October 1997, the drugstore has a working soda fountain and a prescription area on the first floor of the museum. The second floor exhibits a turn-of-the-century physician's office and dentist area. Each section contains appropriate artifacts, fixtures, and equipment donated by professionals.

KENTUCKY

DANVILLE

The McDowell House and Apothecary Shop
125-127 South Second Street
Danville, KY 40422
(606) 236-2804

Owned and operated by the Kentucky State Medical Association as the Cambus-Kenneth Foundation under the Kentucky Medical Association. Carol Senn, curator.

Monday - Saturday	10:00 a.m. - 4:00 p.m.
Sunday	2:00 p.m. - 4:00 p.m.

Admission - adults $5.00; children under 12, $1.00; students 13-21 years old $2.00; senior citizens $3.00.

An authentic restoration to commemorate Dr. Ephraim S. McDowell (1771 - 1830), the father of abdominal surgery who in 1809 was the first to successfully remove an ovarian tumor; he is considered America's most famous frontier physician and surgeon. The original house, apothecary shop, and two gardens were restored through the assistance of the Kentucky Medical Association. McDowell's apothecary shop is believed to have been the first pharmacy west of the Alleghenies. In 1795, Dr. McDowell and a physician partner started medical practice by dispensing medications in the two-room brick building. The front room was used as an apothecary shop continuously until 1856, while the back room was the physician's office.

The restored apothecary shop was furnished and dedicated as a pharmacy museum in 1959 by the Kentucky Pharmaceutical Association. It contains a large collection of late-eighteenth- and early-nineteenth-century apothecary equipment, furnishings, and utensils. These include syrups and extracts, English delft drug jars, Scottish carboys and other glassware, queens ware, English leech and tobacco jars, scales (including an 1842 rare brass Austrian balance), mortars and pestles, and walls lined with 76 gold-labeled drawers with herbs, crude drugs, and chemicals.

HARRODSBURG

Shaker Village of Pleasant Hill
3501 Lexington Road
Harrodsburg, KY 40330
(606) 734-5411

Governed by Shakertown at Pleasant Hill, Inc. Larrie S. Curry, museum director.

April - October
Daily 9:30 a.m. - 5:30 p.m.
November - March
Daily 10:00 a.m. - 4:30 p.m.

Admission - adults \$9.50; youth (12-18) \$5.00; children (6-11) \$3.00; under 6 free.

The Shaker Village features an exhibit of medicinal plants, nineteenth-century equipment, and tools used in the preparation of herbs, and includes other items related to the Shaker pharmaceutical industry. These include drying racks, pill dryers, herb cradle, herb mincer, herb press, screens, sieves, apothecary bottles, pill bottles, distilling equipment, and a press for labeling products. Herb processing demonstrations occur periodically throughout the summer season. A medicinal herb garden is located next to the exhibition building.

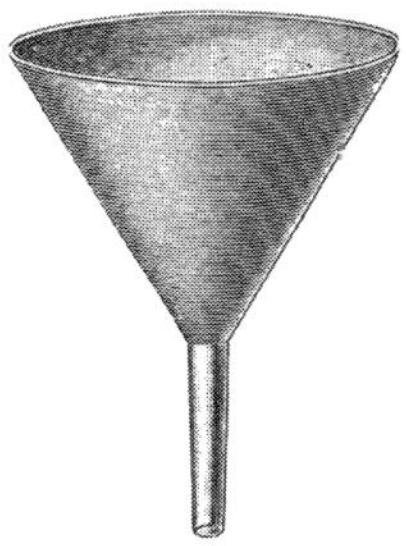

GLASS FUNNELS—Hand Made.

Plain or Fluted. Angle of 60°.

By an arrangement of our own device, we are able to make Chemical Funnels of the correct angle and best shape for preserving the filter paper.

		Per doz.
1 ounce,	2 inches diameter	\$2 15
2 ounce,	2½ inches diameter	2 25
¼ pint,	3½ inches diameter	2 70
½ pint,	4¼ inches diameter	3 50
1 pint,	5½ inches diameter	4 20
1 quart,	7 inches diameter	6 20
½ gallon,	8½ inches diameter	9 60
1 gallon,	10½ inches diameter	15 75
2 gallon,	13 inches diameter	21 50

Ground off at top, when so ordered, at extra price.

For Funnels with Long Stems, see page 67.

LOUISIANA

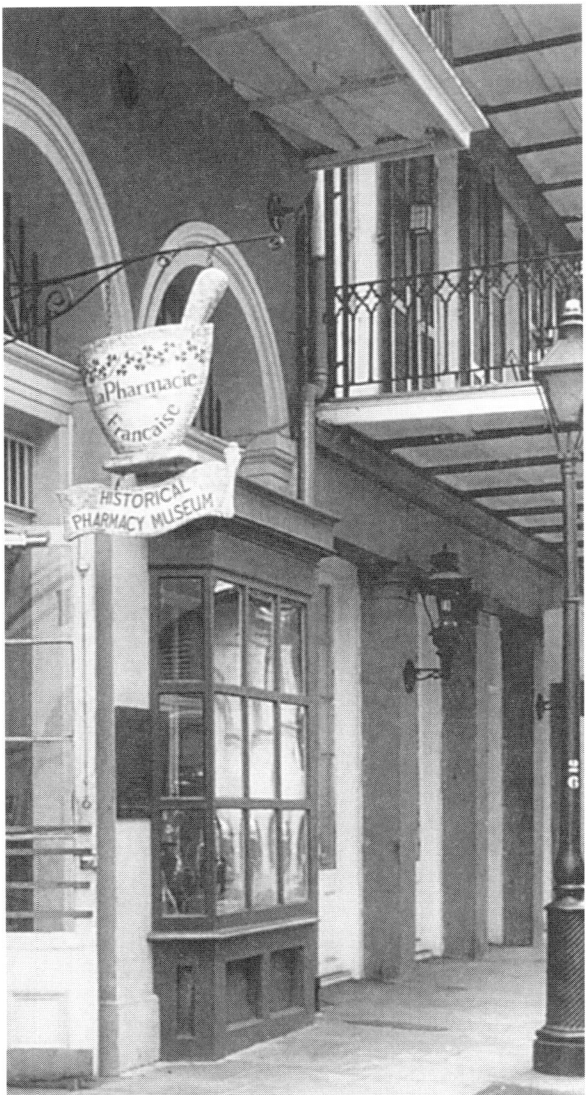

The New Orleans Pharmacy Museum located in the French Quarter.

NEW ORLEANS

New Orleans Pharmacy Museum
514 rue Chartres
New Orleans, LA 70130-2110
(504) 565-8027

Owned and operated by the City of New Orleans and Friends of Historical Pharmacy. Clara Collins Bakar, director.

Tuesday - Saturday 10:00 a.m. - 5:00 p.m.

Admission - $2.00 adults; senior citizens/students $1.00; under 12, free.

This Creole-American townhouse was constructed for the first licensed pharmacist in the United States as his apothecary shop and residence, conveniently located in the heart of the Vieux Carré. Mahogany shelves filled with pharmaceutical artifacts, hand-blown glass bottles, patent medicines, medical instruments, voodoo potions, and crude drugs and herbs fill this museum. Herbs were, and are still grown in the rear walled courtyard. The Pharmacy Museum may be used for tours, business meetings, conferences, lectures, and receptions.

MAINE

NEW GLOUCESTER

The Shaker Museum
707 Shaker Road
New Gloucester, ME 04260
(207) 926-4597

E-mail brooks1@shaker.lib.me.us

Owned and operated by the United Society of Shakers. Leonard L. Brooks, director.

Memorial Day - Columbus Day
Monday - Saturday 10:00 a.m. - 4:30 p.m.

Admission - adults $5.00; children under 12 years $2.00.

This museum, devoted to Shaker artifacts and archives and part of an active Shaker Village, was opened to the public in 1931. Presently it occupies four buildings. The herb garden contains herbs from anise and dandelion to parsley and witch hazel, which are planted, grown, harvested, dried/processed, packed, labeled, and sold nationwide.

The apothecary shop houses an extensive collection of equipment and tools used in drug manufacturing such as kettles, stills, presses, pill makers, percolators, herb cutters, drying racks, grinders, and other utensils, goods, and furnishings made or used by the Shakers. In addition, there is an extensive collection of medicine bottles, packaged herbs and spices, posters, nineteenth-century almanacs, and other archival material.

WATERVILLE

Redington Museum
Waterville Historical Society
64 Silver Street
Waterville, ME 04901
(207) 872-6439

Owned and operated by the Waterville Historical Society. Willard B. Arnold III, president.

Memorial Day - Labor Day
Tuesday - Saturday 10:00 a.m. - 2:00 p.m.

Admission - adults $3.00; children under 12 $2.00.

This two-story wooden house was built in 1824, and donated by the heirs of Asa Redington (a corporal in George Washington's honor guard) to the Waterville Historical Society in 1924. The Apothecary opened in 1976, a replica of a nineteenth-century pharmacy. It includes a mahogany and Tiffany soda fountain and fixtures, a phone booth, prescription ledgers dating back to 1801, medicine and herb containers, drug jars, show globes, show cases, posters, period cabinets and shelving, and tools of the apothecary.

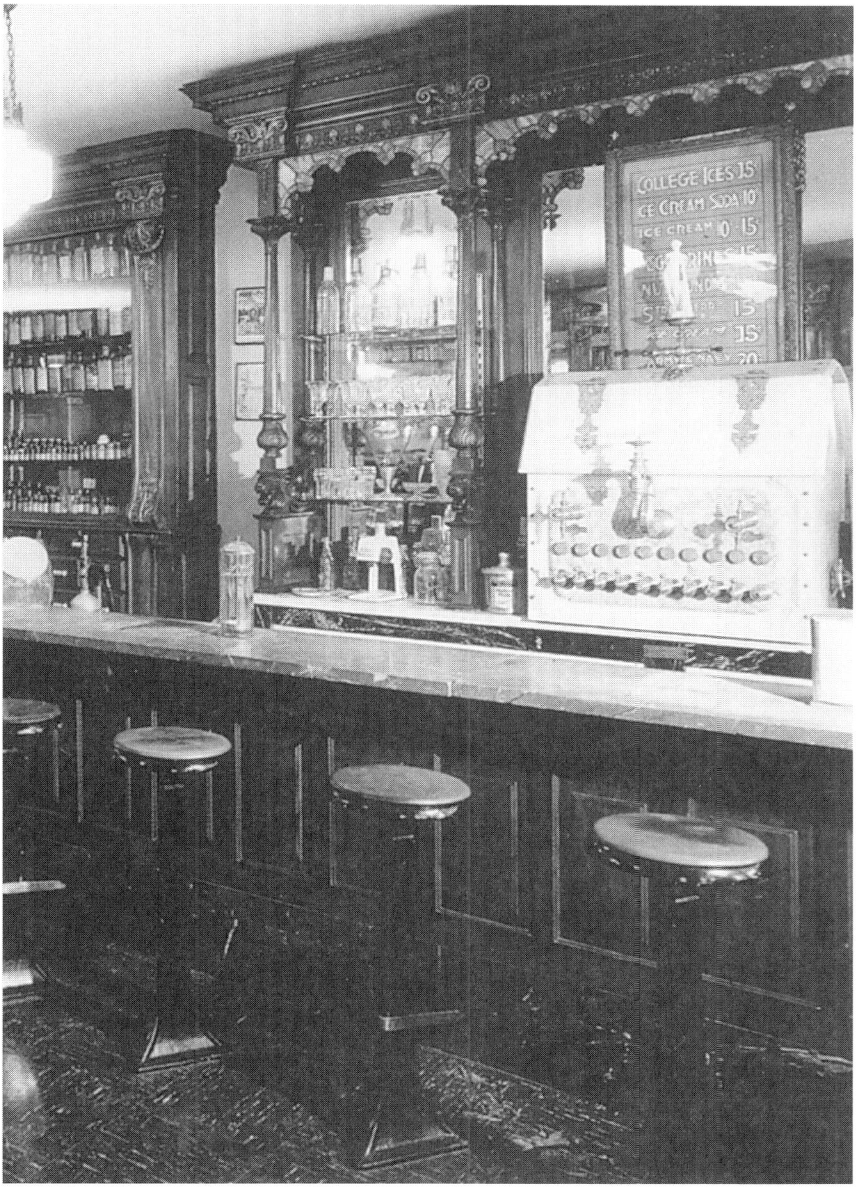
COLLEGE ICES 15
ICE CREAM SODA 10
ICE CREAM 10 · 15

The LaVerdiere Apothecary
Redington Museum of the Waterville Historical Society
Waterville, Maine

MARYLAND

Frederick

National Museum of Civil War Medicine
84 E. Patrick Street
P.O. Box 407
Frederick, MD 21701
(301) 695-1864

E-mail Museum@CivilWarMedicine.org

Governed by the Board of Directors. JaNeen Smith, executive director.

Monday - Sunday 10:00 a.m. - 5:00 p.m.

Admission - adults $2.50; senior citizens $2.00; children 10-16 $1.00; under 10 free.

A museum dedicated to the care and nurturing of wounded soldiers and their medical needs. Exhibited are surgical kits, pharmaceutical items (surgeon's drugcase), and a variety of other related artifacts to the wounded and sick of the Civil War.

Rockville

Food and Drug Administration History Office
Room 13-51
5600 Fishers Lane
Rockville, MD 20857
(301) 443-6367

E-mail jswann@ora.fda.gov

Operated by the Food and Drug Administration. John Swann, historian.

Open by appointment only.

Admission - free

The FDA History Office collects and exhibits drugs, biologics, foods, medical devices, cosmetics, pesticides, colors, and ephemera. Many of these objects were of regulatory interest to the agency, but they all represent commodities that fall under FDA's jurisdiction. In addition, the History Office collection includes equipment used for inspections and analysis of specimens. The exhibit area consists of several display cases distributed among the different components of the agency.

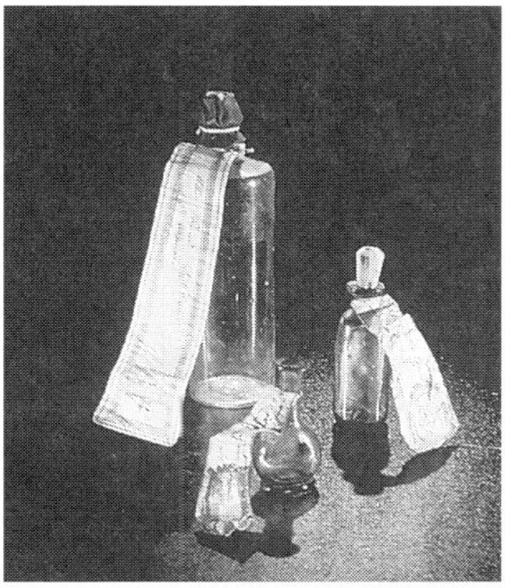

Eighteenth-century drug jars with labels.

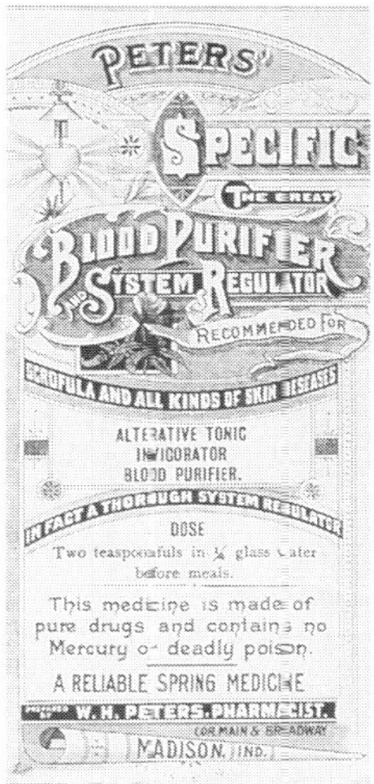

Patent medicines (pre-1906) said little about the contents.

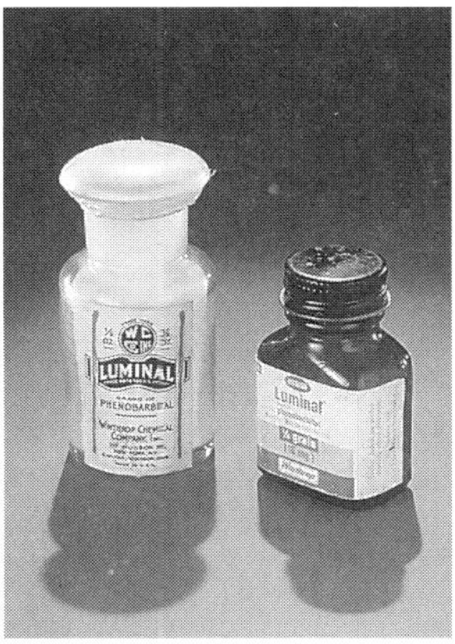

Example of labeling before 1938 and after 1951.

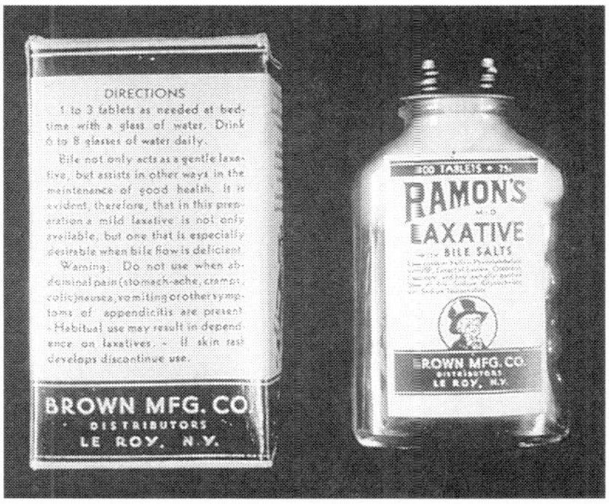

After 1938 products such as Ramons were required to have warnings to consumer.

Artifacts from the collection of the Food and Drug Adminstration History Office, Rockville, Maryland.

MASSACHUSETTS

ABINGTON

Dyer Memorial Library
28 Centre Avenue
P.O. Box 2245
Abington, MA 02351
(781) 878-8480

Owned and operated by the Marietta W. Dyer Memorial Library. Marion Delany, curator.

Tuesday - Friday	1:00 p.m.- 5:00 p.m.
2nd and 4th Saturdays	12:00 p.m. - 4:00 p.m.

Admission - free

Dedicated in 1970 "to those physicians who made their rounds on horseback and to the apothecaries who practiced the curing trade in Old Abington in the good old days." A reconstructed shop inspired in its physical design by the story of Christopher and Charles Marshall of eighteenth-century Philadelphia, as depicted in George A. Bender's *Great Moments in Pharmacy,* painted by Robert Thom.

On exhibit are surgical instruments used by Drs. H.H. Dudley and Gridley Thaxter, ship's surgeon and "physic" during the American Revolution, and Thaxter's son, who practiced at Abington during the horse-and-buggy era.

On display are nineteenth-century pharmaceutical equipment and tools, patent medicines, shelfware, medical kits and saddle bags, dried herbs, glass-labeled tincture and salt-mouth bottles, a marble-topped pan and candy scales, medical and surgical instruments, and prescription registers of Drs. F.L. Bemis (1871 - 1878), J.C. Hovey (1885 - 1888), and C.D. Nash (1914 - 1916).

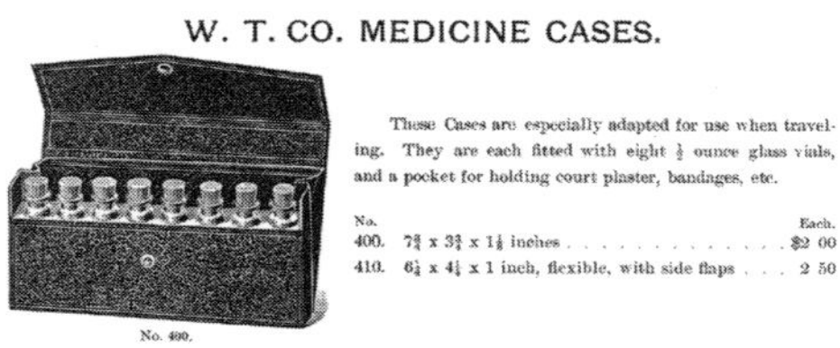

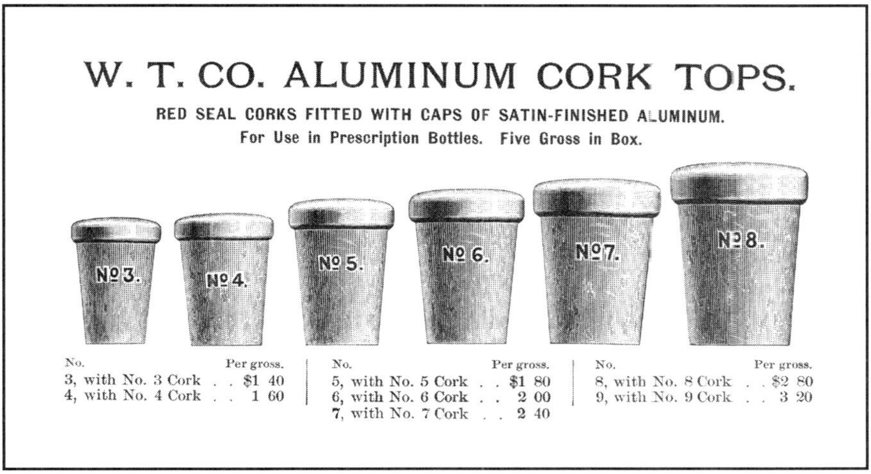

CAMBRIDGE

Botanical Museum of Harvard University
26 Oxford Street
Cambridge, MA 02138
(617) 495-2326

Affiliated with Harvard University. Susan M. Rossi-Wilcox, curatorial associate.

Monday - Saturday	9:00 a.m. - 5:00 p.m.
Sunday	1:00 p.m. - 5:00 p.m.

Admission - adults $5.00; students/senior citizens $4.00; children (3-13) $3.00.

The museum features a research collection of botany specimens including crude drugs and a unique collection of L. and R. Blaschka glass models of plants.

At 22 Divinity Avenue, there is the Harvard University Herberia (telephone: 495-2364) founded at Harvard in 1864; it is devoted to botany with important specimens of flowering plants, gymnosperms, and ferns.

Northborough

Northborough Historical Society
52 Main Street
P.O. Box 661
Northborough, MA 01532
(508) 393-6298

Owned and operated by Northborough Historical Society, Inc. Ellen Racine, curator.

May, June, September and October
Sundays 2:00 p.m. - 4:00 p.m.
All other times by appointment.

Admission - free

A pharmacy display of the late eighteenth century, which includes pharmaceutical tools, saddlebags, scales, and bloodletting instruments used by Stephen Ball, a physician of the Revolutionary period.

Salem

Peabody Essex Museum
East India Square
Salem, MA 01970
(978) 745-9500

Owned and operated by the Peabody Essex Museum. Dan L. Monroe, executive director.

Open by appointment only.

Admission - call for fees.

There is a one-room reconstruction within the seventeenth-century John Ward House (one of the museum's historic properties) of an apothecary shop established in Salem in 1822 by Dr. William Webb. It contains tools and basic equipment of the 1830-1850 period. Also in the collections of the museum are other pharmaceutical items including a bust of Paracelsus (ca. 1840) from the Emerton Apothecary Shop.

MICHIGAN

ALPENA

Jesse Besser Museum
491 Johnson Street
Alpena, MI 49707
(517) 356-2202

E-mail jbmuseum@northland.lib.mi.us

Owned and operated by the Jesse Besser Museum. Dennis R. Bodem, executive director.

Monday - Wednesday, Friday	10:00 a.m.- 5:00 p.m.
Thursday	10:00 a.m. - 9:00 p.m.
Saturday and Sunday	12:00 p.m. - 5:00 p.m.

Admission - family $5.00; adults $2.00; children/students/senior citizens $1.00.

The museum was established by industrialist-benefactor Jesse Besser (1881-1970) and opened to the public in 1966. It is an accredited regional museum illustrating growth in art, history, technology, and the natural sciences. The pharmacy is a store-front window display in the museum's 1890s Avenue of Shops. The exhibit includes numerous pharmaceutical bottles, paraphernalia, and ephemera, as well as an unusual show globe. The pharmacy is one of twelve shops on the avenue.

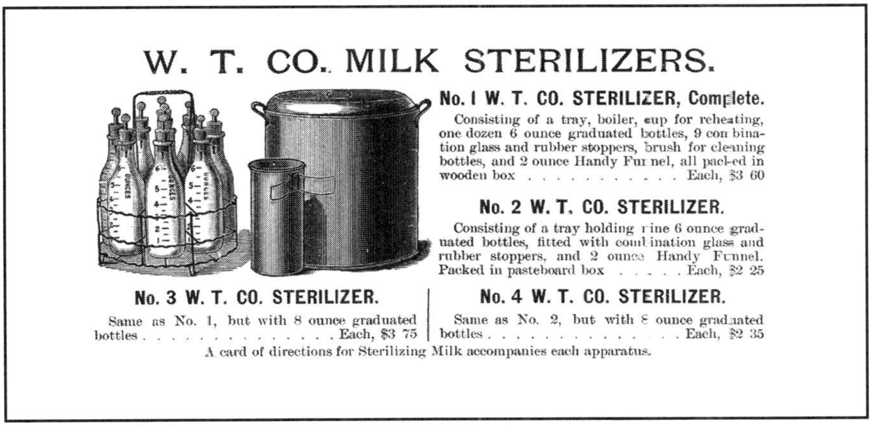

Dearborn

Henry Ford Museum & Greenfield Village
20900 Oakwood Blvd.
Dearborn, MI 48124
(313) 982-6100

E-mail info@hfmgv.org

Owned and operated by the Edison Institute, Inc. Steven K. Hamp, president.

Daily 9:00 a.m. - 5:00 p.m.

Admission - adults $12.50; senior citizens $11.50; children 5-12 $7.25; children under 4 free.

Dedicated to celebrating the spirit of innovation and resourcefulness in America, Henry Ford Museum & Greenfield Village is an indoor/outdoor museum housing over one million three-dimensional artifacts and 25 million paper artifacts. The collections include a large variety of pharmaceutical glassware.

Detroit

Detroit Historical Museum
5401 Woodward at Kirby
Detroit, MI 48202
(313) 833-1805

Owned and operated by the City of Detroit. Maude Lyon, director.

Wednesday - Friday 9:30 a.m. - 5:00 p.m.
Saturday and Sunday 10:00 a.m. - 5:00 p.m.

Admission - adults $3.00; senior citizens and 12 - 17 $1.50; under age 12 are free.

A pharmacy is installed on the ground floor in the "Streets of Old Detroit" at the Detroit Historical Museum. It represents a simulated 1895-1905 pharmacy. This walk-in exhibit displays artifacts and decorative embellishments collected over fifteen years. Dominating the side wall is a massive cabinet made by the Sable Store and Office Furniture Company of Detroit. The drawers are covered with protective galvanized metal, and the shelves are stocked with hand-blown and molded, glass-labeled medicine bottles, proprietary drugs, cosmetic vases, and tin pressed-herb cans. On display also are show globes, an original soda fountain, and an ice-cream table and chairs. In addition, the museum's collection contains 2,000 items from George A. Bender's collection, which exemplifies the growth of Parke, Davis and Company as well as America's pharmaceutical industry.

DETROIT

Pharmuseum
Wayne State University
College of Pharmacy
1400 Chrysler Freeway
Detroit, MI 48201
(313) 577-1574

Owned and operated by Wayne State University College of Pharmacy and Allied Health Professions. Jane Rogan, curator-in-charge.

Open by appointment only.

Admission - free

The collection was donated in 1972 by Howard Mordue, Jr., in memory of his father Howard Mordue, Sr., who was for many years owner of the collection that was imported from Europe. The mahogany fixtures are both French and German. The marble-topped prescription counter is French. Belgian hand-blown jars are displayed. Numerous show globes, both hanging and standing, mortars and pestles, and a set of metal drug canisters are all displayed.

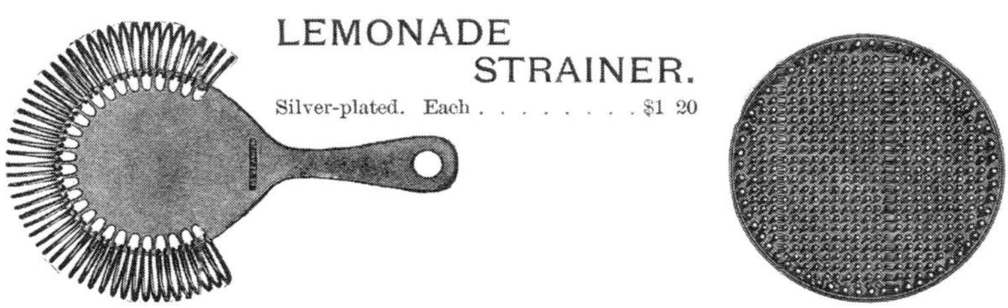

Grand Rapids

Public Museum of Grand Rapids
Van Andel Museum Center
272 Pearl Street. NW
Grand Rapids, MI 49504-5371
(616) 456-3977

E-mail staff@grmuseum.org

Owned and operated by the City of Grand Rapids. Timothy J. Chester, director.

Daily 9:00 a.m. - 5:00 p.m.

Admission - adults $5.00; seniors $4.00; children under 18 $2.00; children under 3 free.

The Public Museum of Grand Rapids was founded in 1854 and now comprises four museums: Van Andel Museum Center, Roger B. Chaffee Planetarium & Veen Observatory, Voight House Victorian Museum, and Blanford Nature Center. There are two principal pharmacy collections. The DeKruif Collection contains early nineteenth-century medical and pharmaceutical material. Most of this collection is not on view. The William Rudell collection preserves the contents of a family run drugstore in Sault Sainte Marie, Michigan, from 1900 until the late 1960s. Over 15,000 items in the collection include show cases and original light fixtures and a cherry-wood prescription counter facade. A later art, and crafts era soda fountain includes an early Coca-Cola ceramic syrup dispenser. The Rudell Drug Store is on display in the Van Andel Museum Center.

Kalamazoo

Kalamazoo Valley Museum
230 North Rose Street
P.O. Box 4070
Kalamazoo, MI 49003-4070
(616) 373-7984

Governed by Kalamazoo Valley Community College. Thomas Dietz, curator of research.

Monday, Tuesday, Thursday and Friday 10:00 a.m. - 6:00 p.m.
Wednesday 10:00 a.m. - 9:00 p.m.
Sunday 1:00 p.m. - 5:00 p.m.

Admission - free

The collection includes a number of pharmaceuticals of the Upjohn Company, a major pharmaceutical company in Kalamazoo for over 100 years.

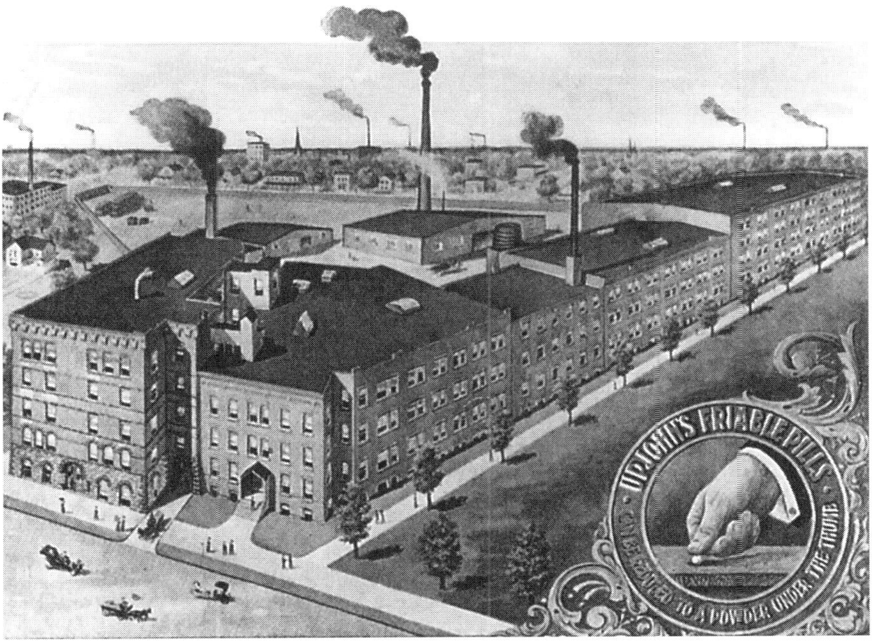

Early Twentieth-century postcard of the Upjohn Company, Kalamazoo, Michigan. Postcard from the collection of Morton S. Fisher.

MANISTEE

Manistee County Historical Society
425 River Street
Manistee, MI 49660
(616) 723-5531

Owned and operated by the Manistee County Historical Society, Inc. Steve Harold, director.

Monday - Saturday 10:00 a.m. - 5:00 p.m.
Closed Mondays October 1- May 31

Admission - $4.00 family; $1.50 per person.

The Manistee County Historical Society is a restoration of the Lyman Drug Company housed from about 1880 to 1957 in a building on Manistee's main business street. It was established and operated by pharmacist A.H. Lyman until his death in 1896. As a wholesale pharmacy, it was the first and only one in Northern Michigan. After Lyman's death, it was purchased by Frank White and Leonard Short. In 1961 the building was given to the Historical Society. It contains a large collection of patent-medicine packages and containers, shelfware, and glass bottles, scales, mortars and pestles, drug grinders and sifters, pill machines, prescription files, a large collection of historical photographs, original posters, and show globes.

MINNESOTA

Grand Rapids

Itasca Heritage Center
10 5th Street, NW
P.O. Box 664
Grand Rapids, MN 55744
(218) 326-6431

Owned and operated by the Itasca County Historical Society. Jodi Maki, executive director.

Monday - Friday 9:30 a.m. - 5:00 p.m.
Saturday 9:30 a.m. - 4:00 p.m.
Sunday (seasonal) 11:00 a.m. - 4:00 p.m.

Admission - adults $4.00; senior citizens $3.00; children 6-12 $2.00; Families $12.00.

The collection was assembled by pharmacist Bernard H. Trygstad and exhibited in 1976 as a Bicentennial project at the museum. This authentic old-time pharmacy is housed in a 30 by 30-foot hall displaying in showcases and oak cabinets and shelves, pharmaceutical equipment, drug jars and bottles, patent medicines, chemicals, botanicals, toiletries, and household items. Among the objects are a cachet device, an 1870 drug mill, a 1910 Eli Lilly crude-drugs identification kit, Glogau's alcohol-gas stove, a Phoenix tank dispenser, 1857 trade tokens for Holloway's pills and ointments, a collection of sixty mortars and pestles, and pharmaceutical text books.

MINNEAPOLIS

Bakken Library and Museum

3537 Zenith Avenue, South
Minneapolis, MN 55416
(612) 927-6508

E-mail ihrig@bakkenmuseum.org

Governed by Board of Directors. Elizabeth Ihrig, curator of books and manuscripts, Ellen Kuhfeld, curator of instruments.

Monday - Friday 9:00 a.m. - 5:00 p.m.

Admission - free

The collection includes books, manuscripts, and instruments documenting the history of electricity and its application to biology and medicine. The collection also contains herbals.

MINNEAPOLIS

Wangensteen Historical Library of Biology & Medicine

University of Minnesota
568 Diehl Hall
505 Essex Street S.E.
Minneapolis, MN 55455
(612) 626-6881

E-mail e-chal@maroon.tc.umm.edu

Owned and operated by the Bio-Medical Library University of Minnesota. Elaine M. Challacombe, curator.

Monday - Friday	8:00 a.m. - 5:00 p.m.

Admission - free

The collection consists of artifacts and pharmaceuticals that have been collected by the College of Pharmacy since its nineteenth-century beginnings. Holdings are uncataloged but sometimes displayed in the Wangensteen's cases in the reception area.

South Saint Paul

Dakota County Historical Society Museum
130 Third Avenue, North
South Saint Paul, MN 55075
(612) 451-6260

Owned and operated by the Dakota County Historical Society.

Tuesday, Wednesday and Friday	9:00 a.m. - 5:00 p.m.
Thursday	9:00 a.m. - 8:00 p.m.
Saturday	10:00 a.m. - 3:00 p.m.

Admission - free (donations gratefully accepted).

This is a small pharmacy restoration in the Dakota County Historical Society Museum. It includes original fixtures containing drawers for herbs and other medicines, elegant apothecary jars, patent medicines, health supplies, and tools of the apothecary for the period of 1840-1920. Other related exhibits include a collection of surgical instruments, a fully equipped optical office, hearing aids, a medical and dental office and equipment, and a barber shop.

STRAW HOLDERS.

FLINT GLASS.

	Per doz.
No. 1	$4 80
No. 2, with Lid	12 00

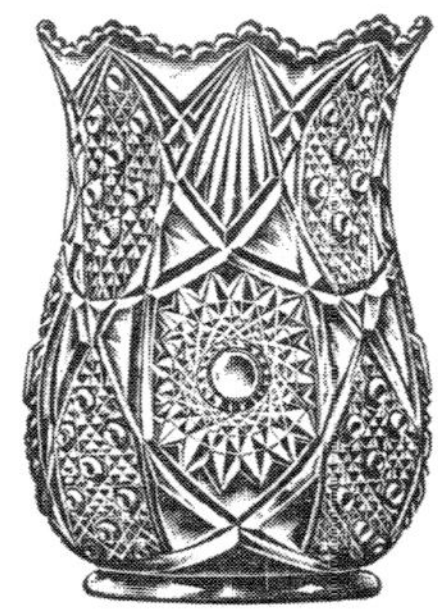

MISSISSIPPI

VICKSBURG

Corner Drug Store
1123 Washington Street
Vicksburg, MS 39180
(601) 636-2756

Owned and operated by Joseph A. Gerache, pharmacist.

Monday - Saturday 8:00 a.m. - 6:00 p.m.

Admission - free

A restoration of a building of the 1860s in the heart of the city's business section, purchased in 1950 and dedicated during the Bicentennial celebration on May 30, 1976. The original structure reminds the viewer of the Civil War era when it was originally built. The collection contains drug jars, mortars and pestles, patent medicines, show globes, medicine bottles embossed with names of pharmacies, hospitals, or name of the drug each contains, and measuring devices, weights, and scales. There are also two antique cash registers, period light fixtures, and a cast-iron gate with a mortar and pestle apothecary sign. This same building houses dental and eye clinics with artifacts.

Adjacent is the Coca-Cola Museum, originally a dry-goods store owned by H. Abraham, who sold it to the Coca-Cola Company, which donated it to the City of Vicksburg for operation and maintenance. In this store, at 1107 Washington Street, the H.H. Biedenharn Candy Company bottled the first carbonated Coca-Cola sold on the market in 1894.

ICE CREAM SODA SPOONS—Silver-plated.

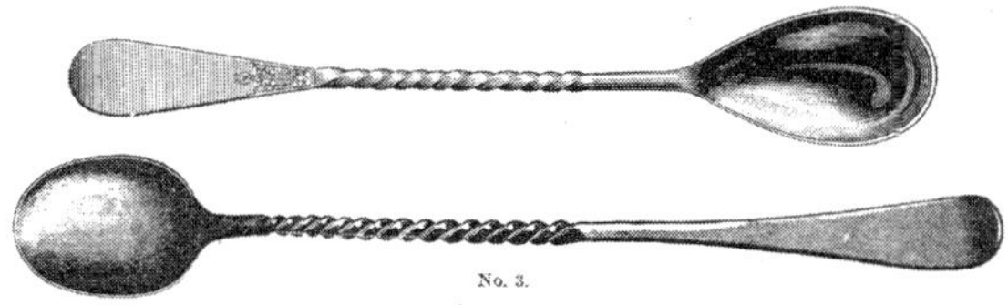

No. 3.

	Per doz.		Per doz.
No. 4. 5¾ inch	$4 00	No. 1. 7 inch. Extra quality	$9 00
No. 5. 7 inch	4 50	No. 2. 8¼ inch. Extra quality	10 00
No. 6. 8¼ inch	5 00	No. 3. 8½ inch. Extra quality. Bowl of Improved Design	10 00
No. 7. 6⅝ inch. Bowl like No. 3	4 50		

MISSOURI

HANNIBAL

Pilaster House/Grant's Drug Store
Southwest Corner of Main and Hill Street
Hannibal, MO 63401
(573) 221-9010

Owned and operated by the Mark Twain Home Foundation. Henry Sweets, director.

Daily call for hours

Admission - free, suggested donation adults $5.00; children (6-12) $2.50.

This two-story house where John M. Clemens, Mark Twain's father, died in 1847 was given to the city (1956) by Mrs. Dulany Mahan. It consists of living quarters with period fixtures and furnishings, kitchen, physician's office, and Dr. Grant's pharmacy. It contains a Fairbank iron scale and pharmacy tools, as well as patent medicines and glass containers from the second half of the nineteenth century. A decorated sign reads, "Prescriptions Accurately Compounded."

The original timbers came from Cincinnati and were brought to Hannibal in 1837 on a steamboat. The building is architecturally one of the most interesting in the city. The Clemens family lived here for a brief period.

POINT LOOKOUT

Ralph Foster Museum
College of the Ozarks
Point Lookout, MO 65726
(417) 334-6411, ext. 3407

Owned and operated by College of the Ozarks. Robert S. Esworthy, director.

April - December
Monday - Saturday 9:00 a.m. - 4:30 p.m.

Admission - adults $4.50; senior citizens $3.50; high school age and under free.

The Ralph Foster Museum includes tools of the apothecary collected by a Springfield pharmacist, Daniel L. Leyerle. Included are early show globes; a large German-made bell-shaped mortar inscribed with the name of the artisan, Heinrich Horst (1657); English creamware leech jar; a pair of amethyst, hand-blown carboys; and a variety of medicinal bottles and artifacts.

St. Louis

St. Louis College of Pharmacy
4588 Parkview Place
St. Louis, MO 63110
(314) 367-8700

E-mail kkirk@slcop.stlcop.edu

Owned and operated by St. Louis College of Pharmacy. Kenneth W. Kirk, dean.

Open weekdays during school hours.

Admission - free

There are several exhibit cases located in the College Library, as well as cases in adjacent buildings, which house the Max Warsaw collection. The collection of fifteenth- to eighteenth-century mortars and pestles and late eighteenth-century Dutch Delft drug and tobacco jars was donated in 1964, and comprises the largest portion of the artifact collection. Other artifacts include numerous show globes, labeled glass apothecary bottles, weights and scales, a tablet triturate mold, percolator, filter stand, spectrophotometer, hydrometers, glycerin pumps, a doctor's pharmaceutical traveling kit and a scarificator. The college also owns a large collection of patent medicines in addition to maintaining a large collection of crude drugs. Many of the apothecary bottles and tobacco jars are displayed in the library inside nineteenth-century pharmacy furnishings, which were originally found in the pharmacy of the Alexian Brothers Hospital in St. Louis.

MONTANA

STEVENSVILLE

Pharmacy of Fr. Anthony Ravalli, S.J.
West End 4th Street
P.O. Box 211
Stevensville, MT 59870
(406) 777-5734

Operated by Historic St. Mary's Mission Inc. Lucylle H. Evans, curator.

April - October
Daily 10:15 a.m. - 4:15 p.m.

Admission - adults $3.00; students $1.00.

The pharmacy, with Montana's first "drive-up" window, is a part of Father Ravalli's log house. On the shelves are many of the original pharmaceutical artifacts including a medicine chest, mortars and pestles, pill board and pill tile, breast pump, apothecary scale, vials, and bottles. Also, there is Father Ravalli's framed prescription for an iron tonic "to be taken with water through a quill." The house is furnished with furniture made by Father Ravalli, together with his books and other artifacts. Restoration is to the 1880 era.

Wedgwood Mortars and Pestles.
"ACME" BRAND.
GUARANTEED ACID PROOF.

No.	Diameter.	Approximate Contents.	Per doz.
0000.	3 inches	3 ounces	$4 30
000.	3¼ inches	3½ ounces	5 10
00.	3½ inches	6 ounces	6 00
0.	4 inches	8 ounces	6 75
1.	4½ inches	10 ounces	7 80
2.	5 inches	¾ pint	10 20
3.	6 inches	1¼ pints	12 00
4.	6½ inches	1¾ pints	15 00
5.	7 inches	2½ pints	19 50
6.	8 inches	3 pints	24 00
7.	8½ inches	4 pints	30 00
8.	9½ inches	7 pints	39 00
9.	10½ inches	9 pints	48 00
10.	12 inches	1½ gallons	54 00
11.	13 inches	2 gallons	63 00
12.	14 inches	2¾ gallons	72 00

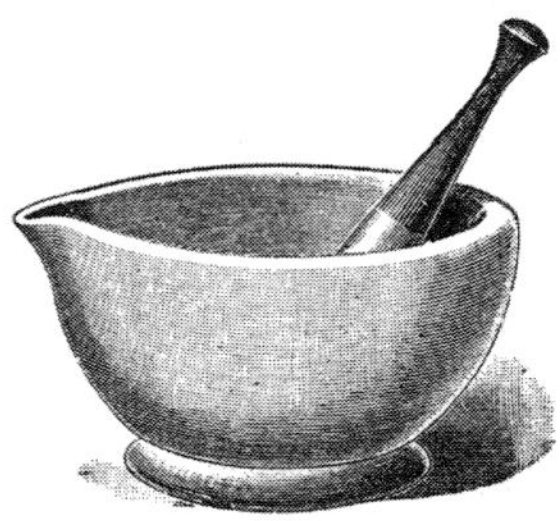

NEW HAMPSHIRE

CANTERBURY

Canterbury Shaker Village
Canterbury, NH 03224
(603) 783-9511

Website www.shakers.org

Scott Swonk, president.

May 1 - October 31
Daily 10:00 a.m. - 5:00 p.m.
April, November, and December
Weekends only

Admission - adults $9.00; children $6.00.

The herb-pharmacy exhibit is located in the Meeting House building, one of the first among twenty buildings in this Shaker village, founded in 1792. It includes herb packages, medicine bottles, vacuum pans, boxes for packaging and shipping of merchandise, pans for making syrups, rack for drying herbs, distilling apparatus, and presses. The Village on 694 acres includes an 1835 infirmary and physic garden.

NEW MEXICO

ALBUQUERQUE

College of Pharmacy
The University of New Mexico
Albuquerque, NM 87131
(505) 272-2461

Owned and operated by the University of New Mexico College of Pharmacy. William M. Hadley, dean.

Open by arrangement with the dean's office.

Admission - free

The pharmacy museum includes a prescription counter and show-cases with pharmaceutical artifacts from the turn of the century. The emphasis is on local and regional history including the history of the college. On display also are objects related to folklore therapeutic agents, especially of southwest Spanish and Indian medicinal herbs and "cures."

NEW YORK

ALBANY

Jabez W. Throop Drug Store
Albany College of Pharmacy
106 New Scotland Avenue
Albany, NY 12208
(518) 445-7212

E-mail bryantb@panther.acp.edu

Owned and operated by the Albany College of Pharmacy. Bobby G. Bryant, interim president and dean.

Monday - Friday 9:00 a.m. - 4:00 p.m.

Admission - free

This is a restoration of the Jabez W. Throop Drug Store of Schoharie. Established in 1800, it continued operation at the same location and in the same family until 1936. It was thereafter moved intact to the Albany College of Pharmacy as an historical museum. The stove, the kerosene oil lamp, the waste-paper container, the ball of twine, the cuspidor, the show globes, and the wooden safe covered with iron sheeting and knobs are all period pieces. The fixtures of pine wood have scrollwork, hand-carved brackets, and labeled drawers with porcelain pulls where herbs and medicines were stored. Other items include patent medicines, circulars, posters, pharmacy registers, glass bottles, artificial nipples, and a period microscope.

BARCLAY PIPETTES.

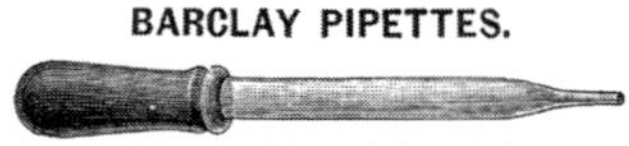

Bent, Straight and Assorted.

1 gross in box . . . . $3 50 per gross.
1 dozen in box . . . . 40 per dozen.

BROOKLYN

Arnold and Marie Schwartz College of Pharmacy
75 DeKalb Avenue at University Plaza
Brooklyn, NY 11201
(212) 330-2700

Owned and operated by Long Island University. Stephen M. Gross, dean.

Monday - Friday	9:00 a.m. - 4:00 p.m.

Admission - free

Exhibit cases installed in the lobby display pharmaceutical tools, glass bottles, patent medicines, and other pharmacy-related memorabilia.

BROOKLYN

The Brooklyn Museum of Art
200 Eastern Parkway
Brooklyn, NY 11238
(718) 638-5000

E-mail bklynmus@rcyonyc.com

Owned and operated by the City of New York. Arnold Lehman, director.

Wednesday - Friday	10:00 a.m. - 5:00 p.m.
Saturday	11:00 a.m. - 9:00 p.m.
Sunday	11:00 a.m. - 6:00 p.m.

Admission - $4.00 suggested contribution.

Collection of sixteenth- to eigthteen- century apothecary jars from Italy and Holland.

BUFFALO

School of Pharmacy Museum
State University of New York at Buffalo
126 Cooke Hall, Amherst Campus
Buffalo, NY 14260
(716) 645-3340

Owned and operated by the State University of New York at Buffalo School of Pharmacy. Ann Triggle, director.

Open weekdays by appointment only.

Admission - free

The Museum was established in September 1986 to commemorate the centennial of the School of Pharmacy at the State University of New York at Buffalo. It reflects the history of the School and the profession of pharmacy. Crude drugs, patent medicines, pharmacy artifacts, pictures, and documents are displayed in the Museum located in Cooke Hall, Amherst Campus. In 1993 a turn-of-the-century Apothecary adjacent to the Museum was created from authentic fixtures and artifacts.

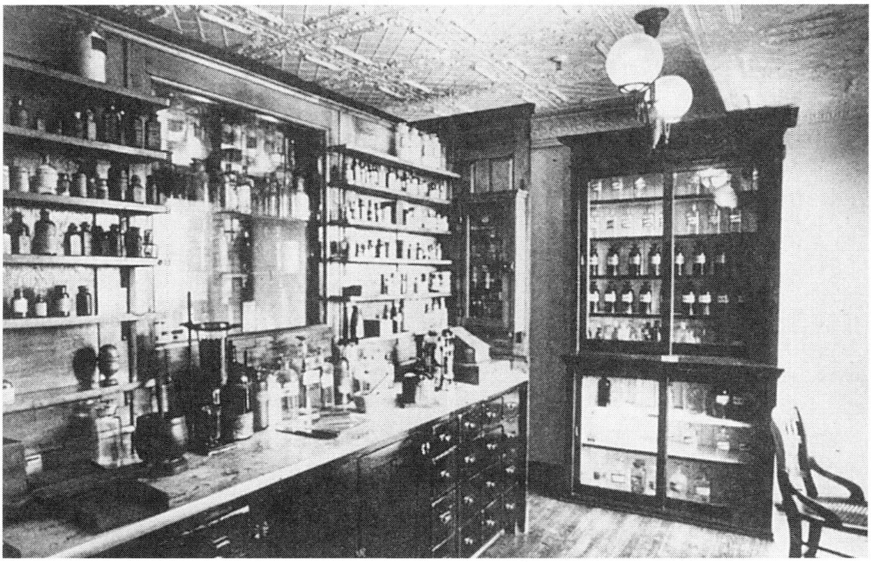

Late nineteenth-century apothecary. School of Pharmacy Museum, State University of New York at Buffalo.

BUFFALO

Buffalo and Erie County Historical Society
25 Nottingham Court
Buffalo, NY 14216
(716) 873-9644

Owned and operated by the Buffalo and Erie County Historical Society. William Siener, director.

Tuesday - Saturday	10:00 a.m. - 5:00 p.m.
Sunday	12:00 p.m. - 5:00 p.m.

Admission - adults $3.50; senior citizens $2.00; children under 12 $1.50; families $7.50.

The Society has in its collection patent medicines, homeopathic medicines, prescription drugs and herbs sold and/or produced in the Buffalo area. The collection contains apothecary tools from area pharmacists. The collection also includes a Buffalo manufactured "Arctic" soda fountain from the pharmacy of C.N. Riggs. Chemicals, extracts, and sundries that were sold at Buffalo area pharmacies are part of the collection. The Historical Society also has in its collections records, photographs, ledgers, and ephemera pertaining to pharmacies that once conducted business in western New York.

COOPERSTOWN

The Farmer's Museum & Village Crossroads
P.O. Box 30
Lake Road
Cooperstown, NY 13326
(607) 547-1450

Owned and operated by the New York State Historical Association. Gilbert Vincent, curator.

KNICKERBOCKER OINTMENT POTS.

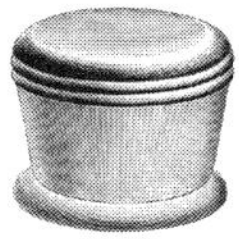

Round Taper Shape. No Shoulders. Inside Corners of Bottom Rounded. Furnished in Opal Glass, with Metal Screw Caps, Brass Finished, Polished, and Lacquered.

No.		Per gross.
1111.	½ ounce	$8 00
1112.	1 ounce	10 25
1113.	2 ounce	14 00

One gross in original package.

April
Tuesday - Sunday 10:00 a.m. - 4:00 p.m.
May
Daily 10:00 a.m. - 4:00 p.m.
June - Labor Day
Tuesday - Sunday 10:00 a.m. - 4:00 p.m.
Call for September-December hours.

Admission - adults $9.00; children (7 - 15) $4.00.

Thralls Pharmacy at the Farmer's Museum is representative of a pre-1845 shop. The building houses a collection of period medicine bottles, boxes and packages, dyes, paints, and cosmetics. In addition, the shop produces a line of cosmetics from period recipies. Next to the shop is a newly renovated specimen garden with over 100 period plants.

The Farmer's Museum and Village Crossroads also includes, a druggist's shop from about 1832. It sold herbal medicines, perfumes, paints, and other sundries. The original fixtures come from Hartwick, New York. Adjacent to it is a doctor's office restored to about 1829, originally from Westford, New York. On the opposite side of the shop, is an herb garden from which the museum staff collects herbs to produce extracts and pills typically made in the nineteenth century.

Corning

The Corning Museum of Glass
One Corning Glass Way
Corning, NY 14830-2253
(607) 974-8220

E-mail cmg@servtech.com
Website www.cmog.org

The Corning Museum of Glass is a non-profit institution chartered by the New York State Board of Regents. David B. Whitehouse, director.

Daily 9:00 a.m. - 5:00 p.m.
Museum will be closed until mid-2000 for reconstruction.

Admission - adults $7.00; senior citizens, $6.00; 6-17 $5.00; under 6 free. Family (two adults with children) $15.00 maximum.

The Corning Museum of Glass is a glass art and history museum with a comprehensive collection of glass vessels, objects, and archaeological remains from every period and area of glass history. About 8,000 objects are on display from ancient Egyptian mummy jewelry to massive contemporary sculpture. Pharmaceutical glassware and other glass from the same period are shown.

MONROE

Museum Village
130 Museum Village Road
Monroe, NY 10950
(914) 782-8247

Governed by the Museum Village Board of Directors. Donald O. Mavros, executive director.

Spring and Fall

Wednesday - Friday	10:00 a.m. - 2:00 p.m.
Saturday and Sunday	11:00 a.m. - 5:00 p.m.
July and August	
Wednesday - Sunday	11:00 a.m. - 5:00 p.m.

Admission - adults $8.00; senior citizens $6.00; children 3-15 $5.00; under 3 free.

The Museum Village has a collection of over 250,000 objects relating the material culture of nineteenth-century rural America. The Charles G. Vernon Apothecary (1886-1948) includes original furnishings, patent medicines, and other merchandise from Mr. Vernon's Drug Store in Florida, New York. Some of the furnishings belonged to the original proprietor, John C. Griddley, who opened the pharmacy in 1840.

CASSEROLES.

PORCELAIN.

No.				Per dozen. With Porcelain Handle.	Per dozen. With Cover and Wood Handle.
00.	(1/8 liter)	1/4 pint,	3½ inches diameter . .	$5 40	$7 60
0.	(1/4 liter)	1/2 pint,	4 inches diameter . .	6 50	8 75
1.	(3/8 liter)	3/4 pint,	4¼ inches diameter . .	7 80	9 60
2.	(1/2 liter)	1 pint,	4½ inches diameter . .	9 60	12 50
3.	(3/4 liter)	1½ pint,	6¼ inches diameter . .	15 25	19 50
4.	(1 liter)	2 pint,	6¾ inches diameter . .	21 60	25 00

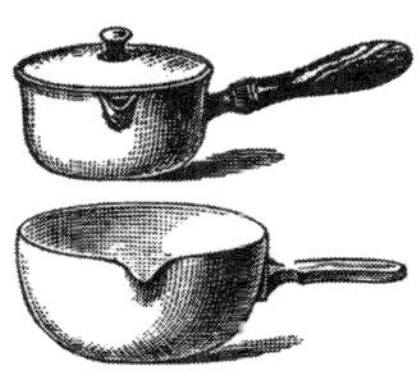

New York City

The Metropolitan Museum of Art
1000 Fifth Avenue
New York, NY 10028
(212) 879-5500

Owned and operated by The Trustees of the Metropolitan Museum of Art. Philippe de Montebello, director. Jessie McNab, curator in charge.

Tuesday - Thursday	9:15 a.m. - 5:15 p.m.
Friday and Saturday	9:15 a.m. - 9:00 p.m.
Sundays	10:00 a.m. - 5:00 p.m.

Admission - suggested contribution $7.00.

The Metropolitan Museum of Art exhibits a representative collection of Italian Renaissance majolica among which are a number of apothecary jars. There are also a few French sixteenth- and seventeenth-, and Dutch eighteenth-century pieces. Important examples of Hispano-Moresque apothecary jars and weights and measures are also included in the collection.

On display at the Cloisters of the Metropolitan Museum of Art, Fort Tryon Park, New York City is another collection of several fine albarellos, examples of Hispano-Moresque lusterware, plates, and deep dishes, principally in the Spanish Room. Inquiries to see the drug pots not on exhibition may be made by letter or telephone.

EVAPORATING DISHES.
PHENIX. PORCELAIN LINED.

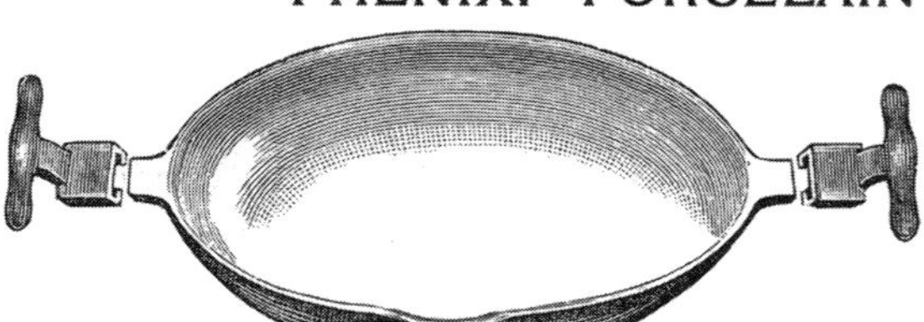

Iron, with Detachable Handles.

			Each.
7 inch.	$1\frac{1}{2}$	pint	$1 00
8 inch.	1	quart	1 20
10 inch.	$\frac{1}{2}$	gallon	1 50
13 inch.	1	gallon	2 20
16 inch.	2	gallon	4 25
18 inch.	3	gallon	5 75

The Porcelain Lining is warranted acid proof, and extends over the oval rim of the dish, preventing the contents from coming in contact with the iron. The dishes are turned smooth on the inside before applying the porcelain, so that the surface of the lining is even and free from holes. Each dish is furnished with two handles, which are easily attached when it is to be removed from the fire.

NEW YORK CITY

Gustave L. and Janet W. Levy Library
Mount Sinai Medical Center
Box 1102
1 Gustave L. Levy Place
Mount Sinai Medical Center
New York, NY 10029
(212) 241-6671

Owned and operated by the Gustave L. and Janet W. Levy Library of the Mount Sinai Medical Center. Lynn Kasner Morgan, director.

Open by appointment only.

Admission - free

The collection consists of twenty-five objects displayed in three cases, given to the Medical Center by Emma Lascoff in memory of her husband, J. Leon Lascoff. Included in the display are a large nineteenth-century counter balance, six mortars and pestles of iron, bronze, and ceramic, ranging from the eighteenth through the twentieth centuries, and a porcelain leech jar.

OLD CHATHAM

The Shaker Museum & Library
88 Shaker Museum Road
Old Chatham, NY 12136
(518) 794-9100

E-mail shakeroldchat@taconic.net

Owned and operated by the Shaker Museum Foundation, Inc. Mary Ellen Hern, executive director.

April - December
Wednesday - Monday 10:00 a.m. - 5:00 p.m.

Admission - adults $8.00; children (8 - 17) $4.00; senior citizens $6.00; children under 8 free.

The Shaker Museum and Library houses over 18,000 Shaker artifacts. Among the twenty-four galleries is a medicine manufacturing room duplicating a room of the "First Family's Medicine Shop" at Mt. Lebanon, New York. Much of the equipment comes from the original shop such as a dried-herb cabinet with four paneled doors. On display are a workbench, power-driven mixing vat, a seed box, Canterbury iron mortar and pestle, a copper alembic, stoneware jugs and jars, and other fixtures built by the Shakers. An herb garden is located on the grounds.

ROCHESTER

Rochester Museum & Science Center
657 East Avenue
Rochester, NY 14607
(716) 271-4320

Owned and operated by the Rochester Museum & Science Center. Eugene Umberger, curator.

Monday - Saturday	9:00 a.m. - 5:00 p.m.
Sunday	12:00 p.m. - 5:00 p.m.

Admission - adults $6.00; senior citizens $5.00; students (K - 12) $3.00; preschool children free.

The museum includes a reconstruction of the William Pierson Pharmacy, founded at Canandaigua, New York, in 1830. The fixtures were installed in 1943 and over the years many artifacts dating from 1860-1910 were added to round out the exhibition. Included are patent medicines (especially those made in the Rochester area), glassware, herbs, grinders, laboratory sink, pitcher pump, show globes, leech and tobacco jars, phrenology head, cosmetics, filters, hearing aids, nursing bottles, eyeglasses, pill machine, splints, scales, mortars and pestles, clock showcases, decanters, and a kerosene lamp.

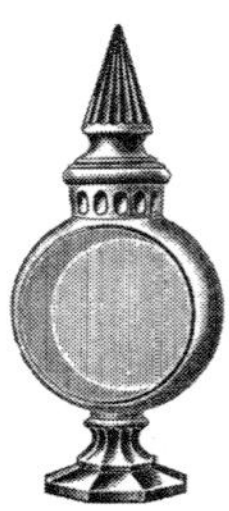

EXPOSITION DISPLAY JARS.

GROUND STOPPER.

No.	Capacity.	Height.	Diameter.	Width.	Per doz.
1	1 quart	14 inches	6 inches	2¾ inches	$14 40
2	3 quarts	18½ inches	8½ inches	4 inches	28 75
3	6½ quarts	23½ inches	11 inches	5 inches	52 50

NORTH CAROLINA

Bailey

The Country Doctor Museum
P. O. Box 34 (Peele Road)
Bailey, NC 27807
(919) 235-4165

Owned and operated by the Country Doctor Museum Foundation.
Josephine E. Newell, curator.

Tuesday - Saturday	10:00 a.m. - 4:00 p.m.
Sunday	2:00 p.m. - 5:00 p.m.

Admission - adults $3.00; senior citizens $2.00; elementary & high school students $1.00.

Founded in 1968, the Country Doctor Museum preserves the medical instruments and tools of pharmacy used by North Carolina country doctors. The Museum is housed in two small restored nineteenth-century physicians' offices moved to Bailey and joined to form a single building. The office of H.F. Freeman, M.D., was built in 1857. The 1884 C.H. Brantley office contains the apothecary shop and physician's office for his practice. Behind the museum is the medicinal herb garden, a replica of the Botanical Garden at Padua, Italy.

Chapel Hill

Patterson's Mill Country Store
Durham County
Route 12, Farrington Road
Chapel Hill, NC 27514
(919) 493-8149

Owned and operated by John and Elsie Booker.

Tuesday - Saturday	10:00 a.m. - 5:30 p.m.
Sunday	2:00 p.m. - 5:30 p.m.

Admission - free

One part of this general country store is devoted to a reconstructed apothecary shop with original counters, shelving, tin herb containers, tools, patent medicines, showcases, a stove, and a variety of posters and other pharmaceutical items. Among the products are Dickerson's Witch Hazel, Bromo-Seltzer for Headache and Lydia Pinkham's Vegetable Compound. Most of the fixtures and artifacts date from about 1900 and include an old-time telephone and cash register, prescription cabinet and files, scales, cork presses, Humphrey cabinet and remedies, and a Munyon's Homeopathic cabinet.

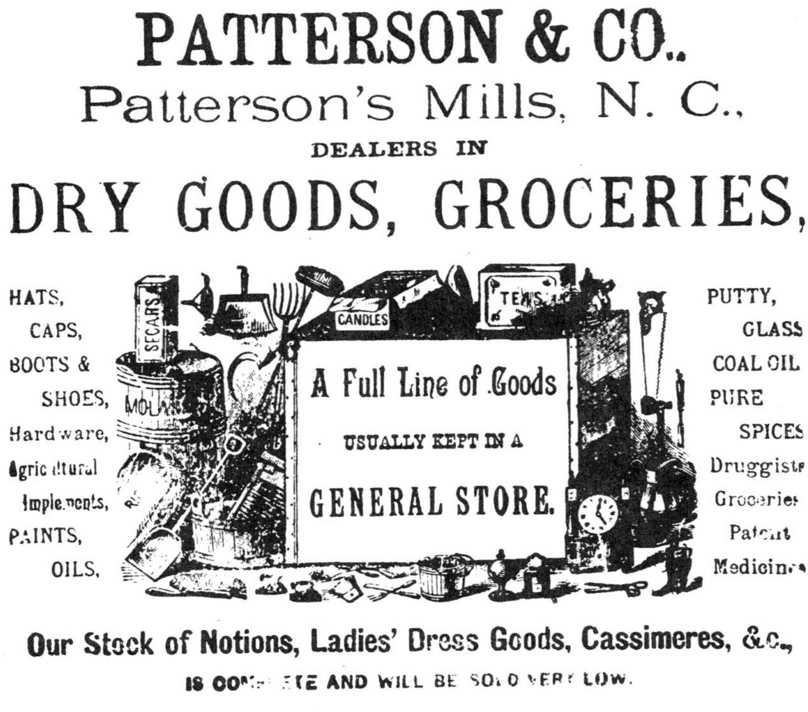

Old advertisement for the original Patterson's Mills Country Store

Patterson's Mill Country Store advertisment (ca. 1870).
Chapel Hill, North Carolina

CHAPEL HILL

University of North Carolina School of Pharmacy
Chapel Hill, NC 27599
(919) 966-1121

Owned and operated by the University of North Carolina School of Pharmacy. William H. Campbell, dean.

Open during school hours

Admission - free

There are several exhibit cases with glass-labeled drug bottles, patent medicines, show globes, scales, mortars, presses, and other tools of the apothecary. The museum was started in 1932 by J. G. Beard, then dean of the school.

DURHAM

History of Medicine Collections
Duke University Medical Center Library
102 Seeley G. Mudd Building
Durham, NC 27710
(919) 660-1144

Owned and operated by Duke University. Suzanne Porter, curator.

Monday - Friday 8:00 a.m. - 5:00 p.m.

Admission - free

The collection contains apothecary jars, wooden cases from an apothecary shop, and portable apothecary bags with drugs intact. There are also a variety of physician's day books with notes about drugs prescribed and compounded.

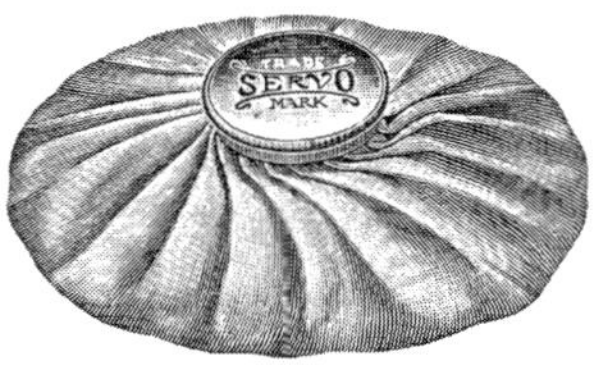

LENOX
SCREW-CAPPED ICE BAG.

SLATE RUBBER, WITH LOOPS FOR TYING DOWN.
FULLY WARRANTED.

9 inch size . . . . $16 00 per dozen

Greensboro

Greensboro Historical Museum
130 Summit Avenue
Greensboro, NC 27401-3004
(336) 373-2043

Operated by the City of Greensboro and the Greensboro Historical Museum, Inc. William J. Moore, director.

Tuesday - Saturday	10:00 a.m. - 5:00 p.m.
Sunday	2:00 p.m. - 5:00 p.m.

Admission - free

The reconstruction of the Porter Drugstore was dedicated as a memorial to pharmacist William Sydney Porter (1862-1910), better known as O. Henry. Here in his hometown, Porter completed his apprenticeship (1879-1881) under the supervision of his uncle, Clark Porter, the pharmacy's owner. The young pharmacist later became a distinguished author. This exhibit includes some of the original fixtures and equipment used in the drugstore.

The Porter Drugstore is also a memorial to Lunsford Richardson, founder of Vick Chemical Company. Mr. Richardson bought the Elm Street pharmacy from Clark Porter in 1890 where he developed an ointment now known as Vicks Vaporub. In 1898 he sold his pharmacy and established the L. Richardson Drug Company, a wholesale house that provided a distribution sale for his remedies. In 1905, Mr. Richardson sold that business and established Vicks Chemical Remedies.

NORTH DAKOTA

West Fargo

Historic Village of Museums
Cass County Historical Society/Bonanzaville
P.O. Box 719
West Fargo, ND 58078
(701) 282-2822/(800) 700-5317

Owned and operated by the Cass County Historical Society. Kathy Anderson, executive director.

Memorial Day- October
Monday - Friday 9:00 a.m. - 5:00 p.m.

Admission - adults $6.00; children (6 - 16) $3.00; Family $16.00.

One of the buildings located in Bonanzaville, U.S.A., is the Prairie Drug Store. Furnishings include a marble top soda fountain, ice-cream tables and chairs, booths for the fountain customers, and all the shelving and counters necessary to complete the interior of the building. Also included are the contents of the pharmacy, which contained many "old time" remedies and patent medicines with names like Dr. Shoop's Croup Syrup, Crazy Water Crystals, Dr. Peter's Magola, Dr. Pierce's Pink Purgative Pellets, Hamlin Wizard Oil Liniment, and Lydia Pinkham's Vegetable Formula. On display are many items used in the manufacture of pills, suppositories, tablets, solutions, and infusions that were a part of the early days of pharmacy.

OHIO

ADA

Pierstorf Pharmacy Museum
Ohio Northern University
Raabe College of Pharmacy
Ada, OH 45810
(419) 772-2277

E-mail t-gossel@onu.edu

Owned and operated by ONU College of Pharmacy. Thomas Gossel, director.

Open by appointment only.

Admission - free

A general collection representing a nineteenth to twentieth-century pharmacy. The main part of the collection is from the Pierstorf Pharmacy of Fairview, Ohio.

CINCINNATI

Cincinnati Medical Heritage Center
University of Cincinnati
Cincinnati, OH 45267
(513) 558-5120

Owned by the University of Cincinnati. Billie Broaddus, director.

Monday - Friday 8:00 a.m. - 5:00 p.m.

Admission- free

A replica of a fifteenth-century Italian pharmacy with over 100 jars is the main attraction. This replica was shown at the 1899 World Exposition in Paris. The collection also contains mortars and pestles, bottles of old medicines, over 500 medical instruments, and an extensive book collection (1700 to present). The museum also holds the original charter of the College of Pharmacy as well as minutes and other ephemera related to the Academy of Pharmacy in Cincinnati.

CLEVELAND

The Dittrick Museum of Medical History
The Cleveland Medical Library Association
11000 Euclid Avenue
Cleveland, OH 44106-1714
(216) 368-3648

E-mail pag4@po.cwru.edu

Owned by the Cleveland Medical Library Association; operated by the College of Arts and Sciences, Case Western Reserve University. Patsy Gerstner, chief curator.

Monday - Friday 10:00 a.m. - 5:00 p.m.

Admission - free

This is primarily a medical museum, but contains several outstanding collections of pharmaceutical antiques. It includes drawers and shelving from the Sterniki Pharmacy (circa 1866); equipment from the

Smithknight Pharmacy (founded 1857); ointment jars from the Petersilge Pharmacy (founded 1881); and other equipment from early Cleveland pharmacies. Also on display are European drug jars, early microscopes, pharmacy bottles, and material related to general hygiene.

COLUMBUS

Ohio's Center of Science & Industry (COSI)
280 East Broad Street
Columbus, OH 43215
(614) 228-2674

E-mail TKessel@compuserve.com

Owned and operated by COSI. Ted Kessel, curator.

Monday - Saturday	10:00 a.m. - 5:00 p.m.
Sunday	1:00 p.m. - 5:30 p.m.

Admission - adults $6.00; students (13-18) $5.00; under 13 $4.00.

The "Durell Street of Yesteryear" at COSI includes an 1864 replica of an American pharmacy with authentic fixtures, shelfware, and tools of the apothecary.

EARTHENWARE BED PANS.

No.		Per doz.
1.	White (see cut below)	$14 00
5.	White	12 00
7.	White, Slipper Shape, with Handle	14 50
10.	Extra Large. Same shape as No. 1	20 00

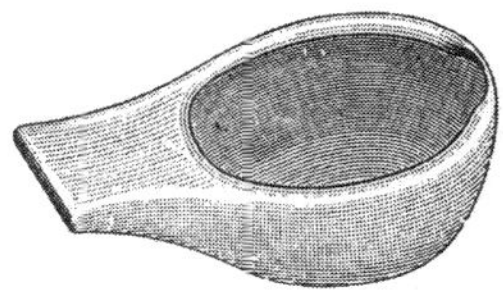

No. 5.

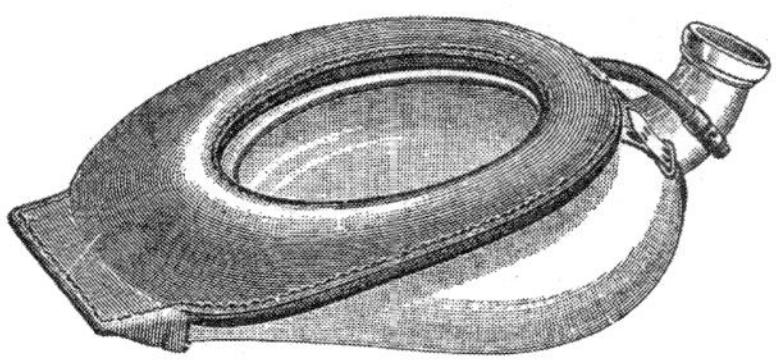

No. 1. Bed Pan, with Cushion.

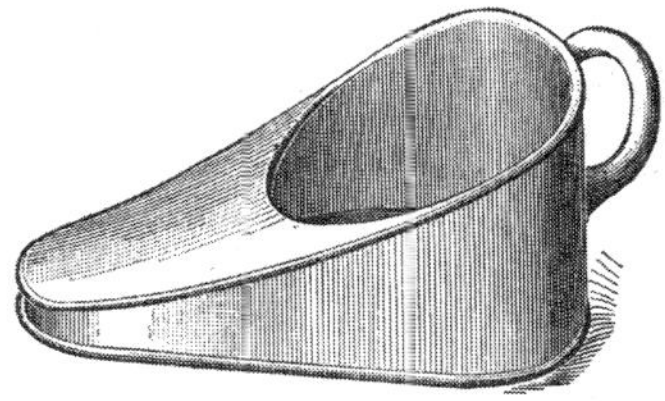

No. 7.

CUSHION FOR BED PAN.

Patented April 5, 1887.

Designed for attachment to an ordinary Earthenware Bed Pan. A Rubber Inflating Air Cushion, of shape to conform to the top of the pan, is held in position by means of a pocket into which the broad end of the pan is inserted, and a strap buckling around the spout, as shown in cut.

Price of Cushions . . . . $30 00 per dozen.

Columbus

Ohio Historical Society/Ohio Village
1982 Velma Avenue
Columbus, OH 43211
(614) 297-2300 General Number
(614) 297-2686 Ohio Village

Owned and operated by the Ohio Historical Society.
Gary Ness, OHS director; Sharon Antle, village manager.

April-November	
Wednesday - Saturday	9:00 a.m. - 5:00 p.m.
Sunday	10:00 a.m. - 5:00 p.m.
December	
Wednesday - Sunday	11:30 a.m. - 8:30 p.m.
January - March	
Saturday	9:00 a.m. - 5:00 p.m.
Sunday	10:00 a.m. - 5:00 p.m.

Admission- adults $5.00; children 6-12 $1.25; children 5 and under free.

The Ohio Village Pharmacy re-creation features the mahogany fixtures built in 1887 for pharmacist Charles Bulfinch of the Hutchinson Drug Company of Lynn, Massachusetts. A portion of the 4,000-item collection of pharmaceutical antiques was assembled by Robert J. Prunchak of Buffalo, New York, a medical service representative for Merrell Dow Pharmaceuticals of Cincinnati, which purchased the collection and donated it to the Ohio Historical Society. The restoration is interpreted on a full-time basis by costumed historical interpreters who demonstrate the preparation of nineteenth-century pharmaceutical remedies.

Hillsboro

Edward B. Ayres Drug Store
114 E. Main Street
Hillsboro, OH 45133
(513) 393-1629

Owned and operated by the Hillcrest Pharmacy, Inc. John Fuller, pharmacist/manager.

Open by appointment only.

Admission - free

American fixtures in 1808 building with many old medicines and artifacts.

Lebanon

Warren County Historical Society Museum
105 South Broadway
Lebanon, OH 45036
(513) 932-1817

Owned and operated by Warren County Historical Society.

Tuesday - Saturday 9:00 a.m. - 4:00 p.m.
Sunday 12:00 p.m. - 4:00 p.m.

Admission - adults $3.00; students $1.00.

This museum on local history and early artifacts from southwestern Ohio houses an extensive collection of early pharmaceutical fixtures, shelfware, patent medicines, herbs, pharmaceutical tools, an 1856 counter, certificates, prescription orders, and filing cabinets.

Tallmadge

Charles R. Weiss Private Collection
637 Ambler Circle
Tallmadge, OH 44278-2401
(330) 633-4342

Owned and operated by Charles R. Weiss.

Open by appointment only.

Admission - free

The collection includes late nineteenth-century and early twentieth-century pharmacy items, drug, and pharmacy trade cards, and almanacs.

OKLAHOMA

Gutherie

Oklahoma Frontier Drugstore Museum
214 West Oklahoma Avenue
Gutherie, OK 73044
(405) 282-1895

Governed by the Oklahoma Pharmacy Heritage Foundation. G. Mark Ekiss, curator.

Tuesday - Saturday	10:00 a.m. - 5:00 p.m.
Sunday	10:00 a.m. - 4:00 p.m.

Admission - free (donations accepted).

Replica of early 1900s drugstore, complete with antique soda fountain. It is the site of the first pharmacy in the Oklahoma territory. The collection contains antique pharmaceutical and medical artifacts.

Lawton

Museum of the Great Plains
Corner of Sixth and Ferris Streets
P.O. Box 68
Lawton, OK 73502
(580) 581-3460

E-mail mgp@sirinet.net

Owned and operated by the Museum of the Great Plains Trust Authority, Drew McDaniels, curator of anthropology and acting director.

Monday - Friday	8:00 a.m. - 5:00 p.m.
Saturday	10:00 a.m. - 5:00 p.m.
Sunday	1:30 p.m. - 5:00 p.m.

Admission - adults $2.00; Children 7-11 $1.00.

Collections include examples of patent medicines of the late 1800s and a recently acquired collection of the contents of a southwestern Oklahoma pharmacy in operation from the 1890s to 1926. Turn-of-the-century exhibits include patent medicines and physician-dentist-pharmacist's office with medical, dental, and apothecary artifacts.

Oklahoma City

University of Oklahoma College of Pharmacy
1110 N. Stonewall Avenue
Oklahoma City, OK 73117
(405) 271-6484

Owned and operated by the University of Oklahoma College of Pharmacy. Rita Pierce, curator.

Monday - Friday 8:00 a.m. - 5:00 p.m.

Admission - free

The exhibition is dedicated to the memory of Lemuel Dorrance, the first graduate of the University of Oklahoma in 1896. The College of Pharmacy and Dorrance Pharmacy Museum were moved from the Norman campus to the University's Health Sciences Center in 1976 and moved again to the current facility in 1983. Focusing on the practice of pharmacy in Oklahoma Territory prior to statehood, the museum displays equipment and tools of the apothecary, drug containers, patent medicines, and fixtures dating from the 1880s to the early 1900s as used in a Territorial pharmacy. Also included is the perfume bottle collection of Dr. Ralph David Bienfang and early laboratory and manufacturing equipment.

Weatherford

School of Pharmacy
Southwestern Oklahoma State University
Weatherford, OK 73096
(580) 774-3760

Operated by Southwestern Oklahoma State University.

Open during school hours.

Admission - free

On exhibit in the School of Pharmacy is a prescription counter and case, books, antique jars, compounding equipment, and pharmacy licenses from the Oklahoma territory.

OREGON

JACKSONVILLE

Southern Oregon Historical Society
Jacksonville Museum of Southern Oregon and
Children's Museum
206 North Fifth Street
Jacksonville, OR 97530
(541) 773-6536

Owned and operated by the Southern Oregon Historical Society. Brad Linder, executive director.

Winter Hours	
Sunday	12:00 p.m. - 5:00 p.m.
Wednesday - Saturday	10:00 a.m. - 5:00 p.m.
Summer Hours	
Monday - Sunday	10:00 a.m. - 5:00 p.m.

Admission - adults $3.00; senior citizens and children $2.00.

Established in 1978, this museum contains a medico-pharmaceutical exhibit with artifacts and tools of the apothecary as well as glassware and patent medicines.

No. 20 CORN CURE BOTTLE.

ALSO ADAPTED FOR DISPENSING TINCTURE OF IODINE.

2 drachm French Square, Flint Glass, with Wood Top and Camel Hair Pencil.

Per gross.
1 gross in Pasteboard Box $9 80

When ordered in lots of 6 gross or more, the bottles can be furnished with customer's name, etc., on one side, without extra expense.

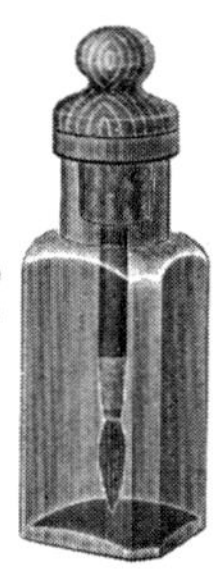

PENNSYLVANIA

BETHLEHEM

1752 Apothecary Shop and Herb Garden Museum
424 Main Street
Bethlehem, PA 18018
(610) 867-0173

Email moravian@itw.com

Governed by the Moravian Museum of Bethlehem; owned by the Bethlehem Area Moravians. Charlene Donchez Mowers, curator.

Individual and group tours by appointment.

Admission - adults $2.00; students $1.00.

Original eighteenth-century fireplace (1752) with equipment and utensils for an alchemy laboratory including retorts, grinders, and scales, as well as Delft jars, glassware, and tools of the apothecary. Adjacent is an apothecary garden, which includes herbs and plants used medicinally by the Moravians in the eighteenth century.

CHELTENHAM

Berman Museum
540 Croyden Road
Cheltenham, PA 19012
(215) 279-2323

Owned and operated by Rosalind Berman.

Open by appointment only.

Admission - groups of 15 or more $50.00.

General store and separate apothecary from the late nineteenth century.

DOYLESTOWN

The Mercer Museum
Bucks County Historical Society
84 South Pine Street
Doylestown, PA 18901
(215) 345-0210

Owned and operated by the Bucks County Historical Society.
Cory M. Amsler, curator.

Monday - Saturday	10:00 a.m. - 5:00 p.m.
Tuesday	10:00 a.m. - 9:00 p.m.
Sunday	12:00 p.m. - 5:00 p.m.

Admission - adults $5.00; youth $1.50; senior citizens $4.50.

Henry Chapman Mercer's (1856-1930) collection of American antiques is assembled here. Included are pharmaceutical and medical equipment collections, medicinal herbs, patent medicines, tools of the apothecary, and dental, surgical, and veterinary implements.

LIGONIER

The Ligonier Apothecary Museum
The Forget-Me-Not Shop
107 W. Loyalhanna Street
Ligonier, PA 15658
(412) 238-6893

Owned and operated by Jacob L. Grimm.

Monday - Saturday	9:00 a.m. - 5:00 p.m.

Admission - free

Prescription furnishings from an 1850 Blairgowrie, Scotland, apothecary shop displaying drugstore collectibles. Also displayed is a collection of free-blown pharmacy glassware.

PHILADELPHIA

Kendig Memorial Museum
Temple University School of Pharmacy
3307 North Broad Street
Philadelphia, PA 19140
(215) 707-4952

Email phamec@astro.temple.edu

Owned and operated by the Temple University School of Pharmacy. Stephen H. Paul, curator.

Open weekdays during school hours.

Admission - free

The museum is dedicated to the memory of Dean H. Evert Kendig who served the school for over forty-two years until his retirement in 1950. It houses a collection of pharmaceutical equipment, shelfware, specie jars, show globes, nursing bottles, mortars and pestles, and other tools of the apothecary. It was open in 1957 and moved to the new Health Sciences Center in 1974. At the entrance the visitor is greeted by two gaslight mortar and pestle signs that are studded with gemlike crystals. The authentic fixtures include an elaborately carved walnut counter and matching shelves, once part of a nineteenth-century Philadelphia pharmacy. The fixtures were originally housed in the Old Morgan Pharmacy where the Wyeth Brothers, founders of the Wyeth Laboratories, had started.

PHILADELPHIA

Marvin Sampson Center for the History of Pharmacy
University of the Sciences in Philadelphia
600 South 43rd Street
Philadelphia, PA 19104-4495
(215) 596-8721

E-mail K.tieger@pcps.edu

Owned by the University of the Sciences in Philadelphia. Kim Tieger, curator.

Monday - Friday 9:00 a.m. - 5:00 p.m.

Admission - free

The museum is located in the first pharmacy school in the United States. The collection includes artifacts and documents relating to the founding of the college; a time line of pharmaceutical development form 1821 (the date of the college's inception); famous alumni who have contributed to the evolution of American pharmacy; the development and changes affecting education in the health sciences; the development of related industries in Philadelphia; and patent medicines. Other artifacts include: mortars and pestles, apothecary jars, medicines, and pharmaceutical equipment.

PHILADELPHIA

The Mutter Museum
College of Physicians of Philadelphia
19 South 22nd Street
Philadelphia, PA 19103
(215) 563-3737

Website www.coll.phyphil.org

Owned and operated by the College of Physicians of Philadelphia. Gretchen Worden, director.

Tuesday - Saturday 10:00 a.m. - 4:00 p.m.

Admission - adults $8.00; senior citizens children 6-18, and students with college ID $4.00.

The museum began as the teaching collection of Dr. Thomas Dent Mutter, professor of surgery at Jefferson Medical College from 1841 to 1856. Today, the museum is housed in the Georgian-style building constructed for the College in 1909. The museum's research collections include diagnostic and surgical instruments, medical equipment primarily from the early nineteenth through the twentieth century, with a few older items such as a seventh-century B.C. Assyrian medical tablet and Greek and Roman instruments. Included are apothecary chests and doctor's bags, patent medicines, pharmaceuticals from the mid-nineteenth century, apothecary jars and bottles, scales and balances, as well as instrumentation relating to every major medical specialty.

Pittsburgh

Elmer H. Grimm Sr. Pharmacy Museum
University of Pittsburgh School of Pharmacy
1104 Salk Hall
Pittsburgh, PA 15261
(412) 647-8494

Website http://pitt.edu/~rxschool
www. lithgow@druginfonet.pharm/~epid.pitt.edu

Owned by the University of Pittsburgh School of Pharmacy.
Jacob L. Grimm, archivist.

Monday - Friday 8:00 a.m. - 6:00 p.m.

Admission - free

Furnishings, prescription medicines, and patent remedies from a western Pennsylvania pharmacy (1900-1940) with an emphasis on University school graduates. A special section pays tribute to ethical drug manufacturers. The Salk polio vaccine was discovered at this location, thus, an exhibit honoring Dr. Jonas Salk will be mounted.

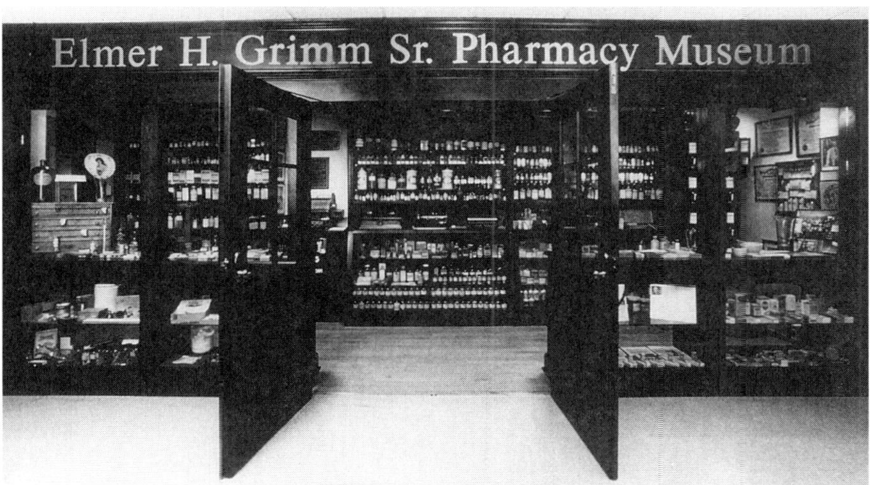

Elmer H. Grimm Sr. Pharmacy Museum
University of Pittsburgh School of Pharmacy.

PUERTO RICO

San Juan

Pharmacy Museum
University of Puerto Rico College of Pharmacy
P.O. Box 365067
San Juan, PR 00936
(787) 758-2525 ext. 5425

Owned and operated by the University of Puerto Rico College of Pharmacy. Ilia Oquendo, dean.

Open weekdays during school hours.

Admission - free

A large exhibition hall is fitted with solid mahogany fixtures, exhibit cases, and dioramas. European drug jars and shelfware are displayed together with crude drug containers, apothecary utensils, a large iron mortar, old microscopes, and archival material. Nearly all the artifacts were used or displayed in pharmacies throughout the island during earlier decades. The most notable single purchase has been the collection of J. Federico Legrand (1858-1928), who also was the first professor of pharmacy at the college. Most of the collection was gathered by Dean Emeritus Luis Torres Diaz, whose personal collection of European drug jars are also on display.

SOUTH CAROLINA

Aiken

Aiken County Historical Museum
433 Newberry Street, SW
Aiken, SC 29801
(803) 642-2015

Operated by Aiken County. Carolyn Miles, director.

Tuesday - Friday	9:30 a.m. - 4:30 p.m.
Saturday and Sunday	2:00 p.m. - 5:00 p.m.

Admission - free

The Henry Moody Drug Store exhibit includes the fixtures and inventory available when it was closed in 1951. It includes a nineteenth-century soda fountain.

CHARLESTON

Charleston Museum
360 Meeting Street
Charleston, SC 29403
(843) 722-2996

Owned and operated by the Charleston Museum. Chris Loeblein, curator of history; John R. Brumgardt, director.

Monday - Saturday	9:00 a.m. - 5:00 p.m.
Sunday	1:00 p.m. - 5:00 p.m.

Admission - adults $6.00; children $3.00.

There is a pharmacy restoration in this oldest museum in the country (founded 1773) to promote natural history and to preserve historical and antiquarian objects. The fixtures are from Charleston pharmacies of the eighteenth and nineteenth centuries. There are medicine bottles, drug containers, herb packages, nursing bottles, medicine kits, show globes, tools of the apothecary, and prescription registers. The two largest collections are the Joshua Lockwood Pharmacy and the Schwettmann Pharmacy, both dating from the nineteenth century.

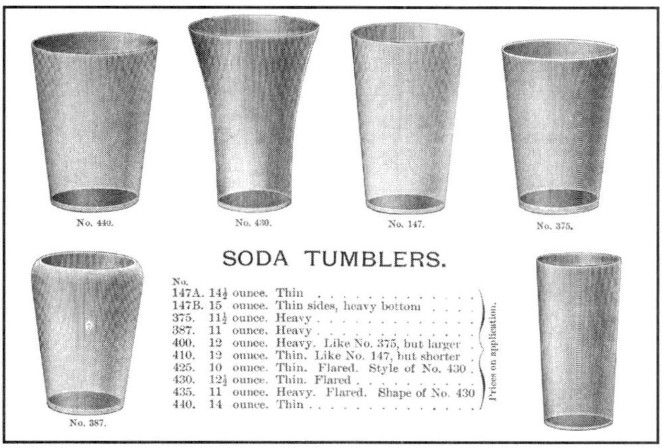
No. 440.
No. 430.
No. 147.
No. 375.
SODA TUMBLERS.
No.
147A. 14½ ounce. Thin
147B. 15 ounce. Thin sides, heavy bottom
375. 11½ ounce. Heavy
387. 11 ounce. Heavy
400. 12 ounce. Heavy. Like No. 375, but larger
410. 12 ounce. Thin. Like No. 147, but shorter
425. 10 ounce. Thin. Flared. Style of No. 430
430. 12½ ounce. Thin. Flared
435. 11 ounce. Heavy. Flared. Shape of No. 430
440. 14 ounce. Thin
Prices on application.
No. 387.

Charleston

Waring Historical Library
Medical University of South Carolina
171 Ashley Avenue, Building 121
Charleston, SC 29425
(864) 792-2288

Owned by the Medical University of South Carolina. W. Curtis Worthington, director, Jane McCutchen Brown, curator.

Monday - Friday 8:30 a.m. - 5:00 p.m.

Admission - free

There are two pharmacy collections on campus. The collection in the Waring Historical Library consists of apothecary jars, medicine bottles, pill rollers, and mortars and pestles. In the College of Pharmacy there is a collection of artifacts reassembling an actual early pharmacy.

Columbia

University of South Carolina
College of Pharmacy
Columbia, SC 29208
(803) 777-4042

E-mail fincher@phar2.pharm.sc.edu

Owned by the University of South Carolina School of Pharmacy. Julian H. Fincher, director.

Open by appointment only.

Admission - free

Artifacts have been collected and are displayed to represent a turn-of-the-century pharmacy. A vintage prescription counter, shelving, and display cases contain 4,000 artifacts, which include tools of the profession, crude drugs, patent remedies, homeopathic remedies, and chemicals. Ice-cream tables and chairs, lighting fixtures, and other nineteenth-century artifacts are displayed.

SOUTH DAKOTA

Huron

H.H. Humphrey & Sons
233 Dakota Street
Huron, SD 57350
(605) 352-4064 or 800-499-4065

Owned and operated by Ralph and Bonnie Gosch.

Monday - Friday	8:30 a.m. - 6:00 p.m.
Saturday	8:30 a.m. - 5:00 p.m.

Admission - free

Visitors can see a photo collection and artifacts from the Humphrey family who owned the pharmacy since 1903. Some of the original decor and fixtures are from the original pharmacy in Wallace, South Dakota. There are also autographed photographs from the Kennedy-Johnson presidential administration. Other artifacts include prescription files, correspondence, a book that contains original directions for compounding, bottles, weights and scales, and mortars and pestles.

Wall

Wall Drug Apothecary Shoppe & Pharmacy Museum
510 Main Street
Wall, SD 57790
(605) 279-2175

E-mail walldrug@gwtc.net

Owned and operated Bill Hustead.

Summer months
Daily 6:30 a.m. - 9:30 p.m.
Closed November 15 - April 1.

Admission - free

Fashioned after the original pharmacy that was located across the street from the present location and founded in 1931, the collection includes over 400 pharmaceutical artifacts.

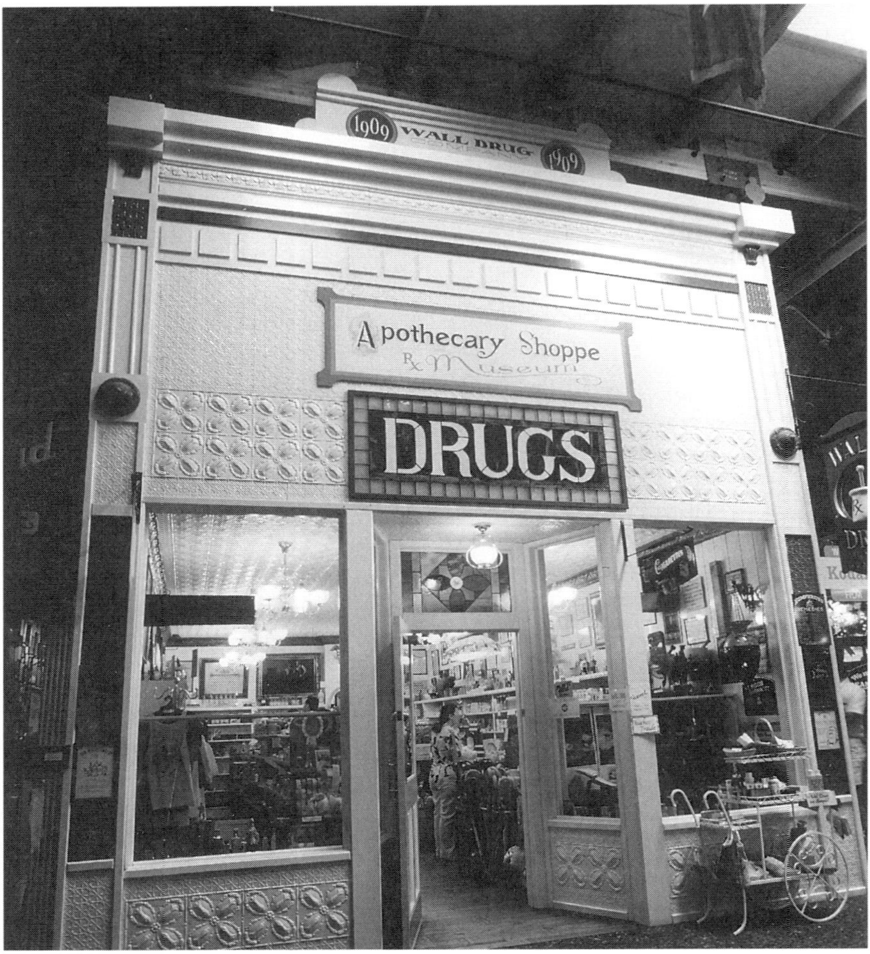

Apothecary Shoppe and Pharmacy Museum at the Mall of Wall Drug Store, Wall, South Dakota.

TENNESSEE

Memphis

Memphis Pink Palace Museum
3050 Central Avenue
Memphis, TN 38111
(901) 320-6322

Email rbristr@memphis.magibox.net

Owned by the University of Tennessee College of Pharmacy and on loan to the museum for twenty years. The museum is owned and operated by the Memphis Park Commission and Memphis Museum, Inc. Ronald C. Brister, collections manager.

Tuesday - Thursday	9:00 a.m. - 5:00 p.m.
Friday, Saturday	9:00 a.m. - 10:00 p.m.
Sunday	1:00 p.m. - 5:00 p.m.

Admission - adults $1.00; senior citizens, children/students $0.75.

Pharmacist Ralph E. Julian (1886-1975) of Morristown, gathered the collection, which was transferred to this museum (founded 1928) after his death. It was first opened to the public in 1930 as a museum of natural and cultural history and after recent remodeling, it was reopened in 1977. Original fixtures and showcases of the turn of the century, as well as show globes, drug jars, patent medicines, a telephone, and a cash register are on display. It contains Coca-Cola accessories, as well as Orange Crush, Grape Smash, and Hire's Root Beer dispensing apparatus. Also on display are tools of the apothecary, a clock, posters, brass light fixtures, herb drawers, and drug percolating and grinding equipment.

MARVEL
FOUNTAIN SYRINGES.

THREE HARD RUBBER PIPES.

A Popular Low Priced Fountain Syringe of Good Quality.

In Paper Box, with Handsome Label.

		Per doz.
No. 3.	2 quart	$14 00
No. 4.	3 quart	17 00

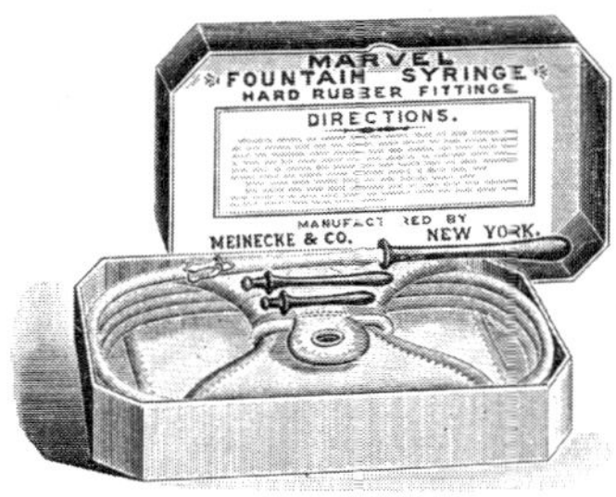

TEXAS

Amarillo

The Texas Pharmacy Museum
Texas Tech School of Pharmacy
1300 S. Coulter
Amarillo, TX 79106
(806) 356-4014

Owned by the Texas Tech University Foundation. Billy Walker, director.

Monday - Friday 10:00 a.m. - 4:00 p.m.

Admission - free

The exhibit includes four large rooms of displays including tools, drugs from an old pharmacy, and an honor room for the pioneers of early Texas pharmacy. Other exhibits include an herb collection, an old post office, pharmacy jars, show globes, scales and balances, and mortars and pestles.

Dallas

University of Texas Southwestern
Medical Center at Dallas
5323 Harry Hines Blvd.
Dallas, TX 75235
(214) 648-2022

Owned and operated by the University of Texas Southwestern Medical Center at Dallas.

Open by appointment only.

Admission - free

Several cases feature displays of drug jars, microscopes, dental, medical, and surgical instruments, medical kits, medical books, prints and graphs; as well as some tools of the apothecary.

GALVESTON

Blocker History of Medicine Collections
Moody Medical Library
9th and Market Street
Galveston, TX 77555-1035
(409) 772-2397

E-mail ref@utmb.edu

Owned by the University of Texas Medical Branch. Sarita Oertling, collections manager.

Monday - Friday 8:00 a.m. - 5:00 p.m.

Admission - free

The pharmaceutical collection housed in the Moody Medical Library consists of assorted medicine chests and cases (nineteenth-century) and non-prescription drugs from the first part of the twentieth century. The mahogany chests with brass handles, intricate compartments, and hand-blown medicine bottles provide a glimpse of nineteenth-century therapeutics. The non-prescription drugs include items manufactured by 368 different pharmaceutical companies in 35 different states. A computer database for the non-prescription drugs can be queried to find different types of information about therapeutics and the drug industry during the first part of the twentieth century. Nearly 40 percent of the drugs in the collection include accompanying prospectuses.

HOUSTON

Professional Compounding Centers of America, Inc.
99012 S. Wilcrest
Houston, TX 77099
(281) 933-6948

E-mail lawson@thecompounders.com

Owned by Professional Compounding Centers of America Inc. Lawson Kloesel, director.

Open by appointment only.

Admission - free

View a compounding museum housed at the Professional Compounding Centers of America, Inc., a company serving independent, compounding pharmacists who provide problem-solving services in a community practice setting. See examples of antique weights, measures, and balances, as well as an early ointment mill, and old fashioned prescription bottles with labels under glass. The collection also features an 1890 dispensing counter, fully restored to its original turn-of-the-century condition.

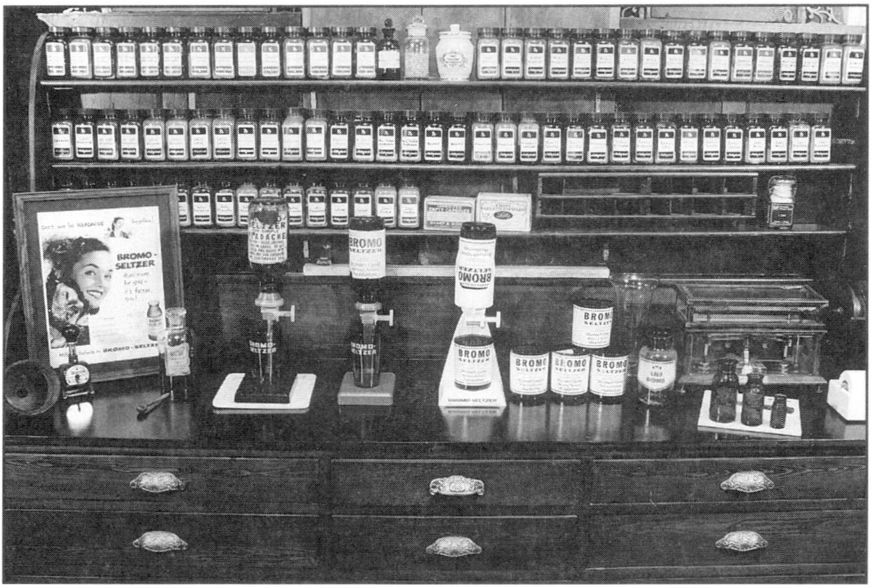

Bromo-Seltzer display at the Pharmacy Compounding Museum Houston, Texas.

JEFFERSON

Jefferson Historical Society and Museum
223 West Austin Street
Jefferson, TX 75657
(903) 665-2775

Owned and operated by the Jefferson Historical Society, Inc. E. P. Storie, director.

Daily 9:30 a.m. - 5:00 p.m.

Admission - adults $2.00; students under 12 $.50.

On display is a showcase with medical instruments and pharmaceutical tools and drug containers. The museum was founded in 1948 in an 1888 post office and courthouse.

San Antonio

Institute of Texan Cultures
801 S. Bowie Street
San Antonio, TX 78205
(210) 458-2300

The University of Texas at San Antonio. Rex H. Ball, executive director.

Tuesday - Sunday 9:00 a.m. - 5:00 p.m.

Admission - adults $4.00; senior citizens; children 3-12 $2.00.

Exhibits represent twenty-seven ethnic and cultural groups with Texan heritage and include a medico-pharmaceutical display. It contains artifacts and illustrations of frontier medical practice and an early Texas apothecary restoration of fixtures, tools, and pharmaceutical vessels and glassware.

Waco

Dr. Pepper Museum & Free Enterprise Institute
300 S. 5th Street
Waco, TX 76701
(254) 757-1025

E-mail joec@drpeppermuseum.com

Operated by the Dr. Pepper Museum & Free Enterprise Board of Directors. Joe Cavanaugh, director.

Monday - Saturday 10:00 a.m. - 4:00 p.m.
Sunday 12:00 p.m. - 4:00 p.m.
Extended summer hours Memorial Day - Labor Day

Admission - adults $4.00; senior citizens $3.50; students $2.00.

The museum is housed in the 1906 bottling factory of the Dr. Pepper Company. Exhibits include "Soda Pop: From Fountain to Bottled Pop," a recreation of Waco's Old Corner Drugstore where Dr. Pepper was invented. The ground floor is dedicated to telling how soft drinks are manufactured and bottled. The second floor tells the story of marketing and advertising and includes vending machines and standing cases. The museum is not part of the Dr. Pepper/Seven-Up Co.

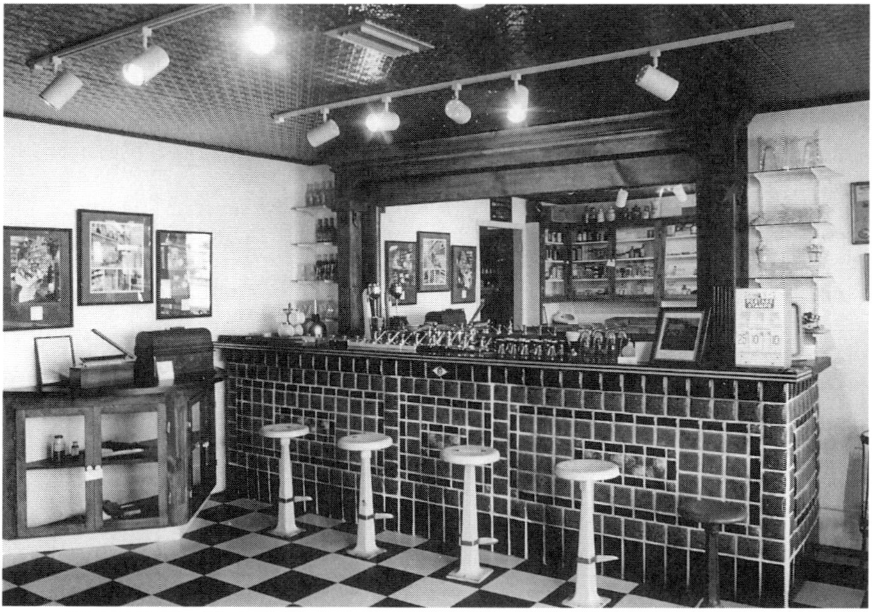

Old-fashioned soda fountain on display at the Pharmacy Museum
Heritage Society Museum of Weimar, Inc.

WEIMAR

Pharmacy Museum
The Heritage Society Museum of Weimar, Inc.
125 East Main Street
Weimar, TX 78962
(409) 725-8203

E-mail lawson@neosoft.com

Owned by the Heritage Society Museum of Weimar, Inc. Lawson Kloesel, director.

Wednesday and Saturday 10:00 a.m. - 4:00 p.m.

Admission - free (donations accepted)

Journey back to the olden days of pharmacy via the Heritage Society's pharmacy museum, featuring more than 2,500 antique pharmaceutical items. The exhibit includes pharmaceutical weights and measures, balances, tools, patent medicines, glass bottles, show globes, archival material, reconstructed fixtures, as well as mortars and pestles. Additional highlights include an old-fashioned soda fountain complete with fountain accessories, back bar, mirror, and cigar memorabilia. The fountain featuring a beautiful tile design, was once located in a Farmer's Drug Store, and has been carefully reconstructed to its original condition. The Museum also features a physician's office complete with period equipment and tools, medicine bags, examining table, and surgical instruments.

UTAH

FARMINGTON

Pioneer Village
Lagoon Amusement Park
375 North Lagoon Drive
Farmington, UT 84025
(801) 451-8000

Owned by the Lagoon Amusement Park. Howard Freed, director.

Call for hours.

Admission - $15.00.

This pioneer village of late nineteenth-century Utah contains thirty-six buildings. One is a reconstruction of the 1893 pharmacy of G.P. Crabtree of Cairo, Illinois. In addition to original fixtures, equipment, and shelf ware, it displays tools of the apothecary, medicine bottles, drug jars, and posters.

VERMONT

SHELBURNE

Shelburne Museum
U.S. Route 7
Shelburne, VT 05482
(802) 985-3346

Operated by Shelburne Museum. Hope Alswang, president.

Late May - late October
Daily 10:00 a.m. - 5:00 p.m.

Admission - call for fees.

Restoration of a pharmacy in operation between 1870 and 1900. The installation includes authentic fixtures and shelfware, dried herbs, spices, drugs, labeled glass apothecary bottles, patent medicines, medical equipment, cosmetics, a collection of barber's razors, and a compounding room.

VIRGIN ISLANDS

CHRISTIANSTED

Christiansted Apothecary Shop
Queens Cross and Company Streets
Christiansted, St. Croix
US Virgin Islands 00820
(340) 772-0598

Governed by the St. Croix Landmarks Society. George Tyson, director.

Monday - Saturday 10:00 a.m. - 4:00 p.m.

Admission - free

The Christiansted Apothecary Shop has been set up in its original location at Queens Cross and Company Street, and is the only Danish pharmacy restoration in the Western Hemisphere. Established by Danish pharmacist, Peder Eggert Benzon, the pharmacy opened in 1828 in its present location, operating continuously until 1970. The pharmacy museum contains the drug jars, pharmaceutical equipment and pharmacy records located in a Caribbean outpost.

VIRGINIA

ALEXANDRIA

Stabler-Leadbeater Apothecary Museum
105-107 South Fairfax Street
Alexandria, VA 22314
(703) 836-3713

Managed and operated by the Stabler Leadbeater Apothecary Museum, Inc. Sarah Becker, director.

Monday - Saturday 10:00 a.m. - 4:00 p.m.

Admission - adults, $2.50; students $2.00.

The apothecary shop was founded by Edward Stabler in 1792: his son-in-law John Leadbeater assumed proprietorship in 1852 and the pharmacy remained in the same family until it closed in 1933. All hand-blown glass tincture and salt-mouth bottles with either gold-leaf or glass labels are from the original pharmacy, which opened as a museum in 1939. Tools of the apothecary include mortars and pestles, pill machines, powder paper folders, and suppository molds. Other supplies that were sold in the pharmacy include eyeglasses, nursing bottles, lancets for bleeding, medicine chests, and medicines. Show globes are displayed in the front windows, and the second floor of the shop includes hundreds of wooden drawers filled with original botanicals and chemicals, and thousands of product labels for the medicinals that the firm produced in the late nineteenth century. Also on the second floor are the archives, consisting of pharmacy records from 1792 until 1933.

Fredericksburg

Hugh Mercer Apothecary Shop
1020 Caroline Street
Fredericksburg, VA 22401
(703) 373-3362

Property of the Association for the Preservation of Virginia Antiquities. Genevieve Bugay, manager.

March - November
Daily 9:00 a.m. - 5:00 p.m.
December - February
Daily 10:00 a.m. - 4:00 p.m.

Admission - adults $4.00; children $1.50.

Dr. Hugh Mercer graduated in medicine from Aberdeen University Medical College in 1744, and migrated to this country in 1746. He entered the Revolutionary Army in 1776 as brigadier general and gave his life on the battlefield a year later at Princeton, New Jersey. Dr. Mercer operated an apothecary shop with a medical office and surgery adjoining in Fredericksburg from 1761 until he entered the army fifteen years later. On display are period pharmacy equipment, faded prescription orders, and yellow-leaved ledgers, books, gold-labeled bottles, and old showcases. Preserved archival materials include accounts written for George Washington.

Williamsburg

Pasteur & Galt Apothecary Shop
Colonial Williamsburg Foundation
Williamsburg, VA 23187-1776
(757) 565-8675

Administered by the Colonial Williamsburg Foundation. Bill White, director, Robin Kipps, site supervisor.

Call 1-800-HISTORY for current operating hours and tickets prices.

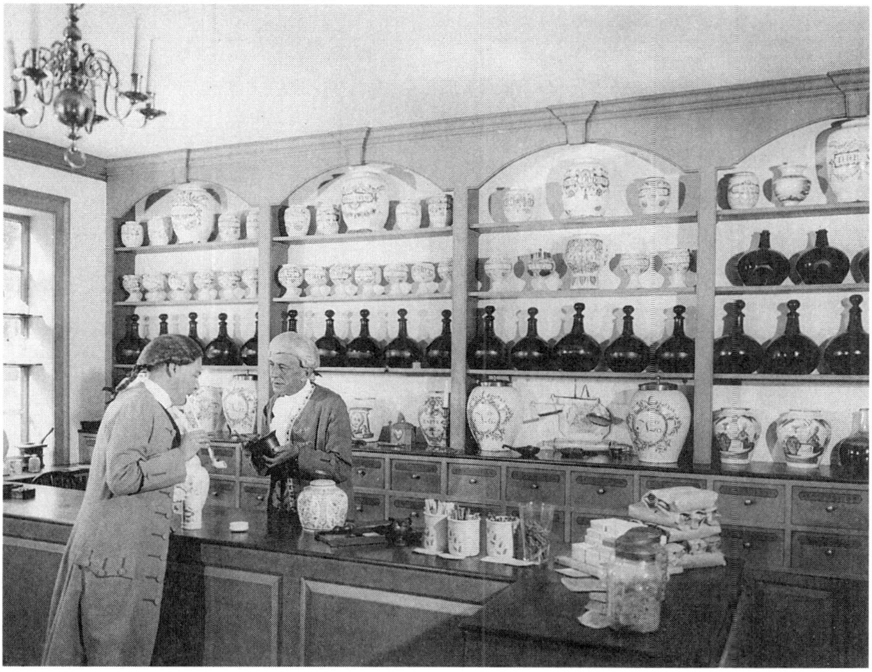

Pasteur-Galt Apothecary Shop, Colonial Williamsburg restoration, Williamsburg, Virginia.

Among the eighty-eight original preserved and over 400 reconstructed historic buildings (dates ranging from 1693-1837) is an apothecary shop reconstructed on the original site. It was opened during the observance of "Pharmacy Week" in 1950. The site features a large collection of original Delft drug jars. Over the entrance hangs a sign featuring a combination mortar and pestle and staff of Aesculapius, representative of the healing arts of pharmacy and medicine. The shop is named in memory of two apothecary-surgeons who practiced on the site. The first is William J. Pasteur. After the completion of his apprenticeship with Dr. George Gilmer (practiced 1731-1757), he was educated at St. Thomas' Hospital in London. He established his practice here when he returned in 1759.

The second is John Minson Galt, who apprenticed to Pasteur before completing his medical education. In 1769 he started his practice in Williamsburg and later served as a partner of Dr. Pasteur from 1775 to 1778.

Winchester

Dunn Family Museum and Archives
Shenandoah University
School of Pharmacy
1460 University Lane
Winchester, VA 22601
(504) 665-1282

Owned and operated by Shenandoah University School of Pharmacy. Alan McKay, dean.

Open weekdays during school hours.

Admission - free

The museum and archives were opened in June 1997 by benefactors Bernard and Anne Marie Dunn. The museum is located adjacent to the Dean's office, while the archives are located in the School of Pharmacy library. The museum features the fixtures of a Sheperdstown, West Virginia, apothecary shop variously operated as Reinhardt's Pharmacy from the 1890s to 1914 when it changed ownership, as Owens & Miller for a time, and then by Hiram Owens. An Arctic Cottage Soda Fountain is also on display. The archives comprises the records of the Winchester Apothecary Shop, including an 1861 account book recording sales to the "Confederate Southern Army," and dozens of handwritten account books from 1808 to 1945 over which have been pasted prescription orders from 1850 to the 1890s. Products sold by the Miller Drugstore are also exhibited.

WASHINGTON

Wapato

Red Cross Drugstore Museum
105 E. Third Street
Wapato, WA 98951
(509) 877-2707

E-mail RCOLE 36615@aol.com

Owned and operated by Bill and Rose Coleman.

Monday - Saturday (call for Drugstore hours)

Admission- free

Complete old-time pharmacy with all prescriptions from 1940 and business records from 1930 to the present.

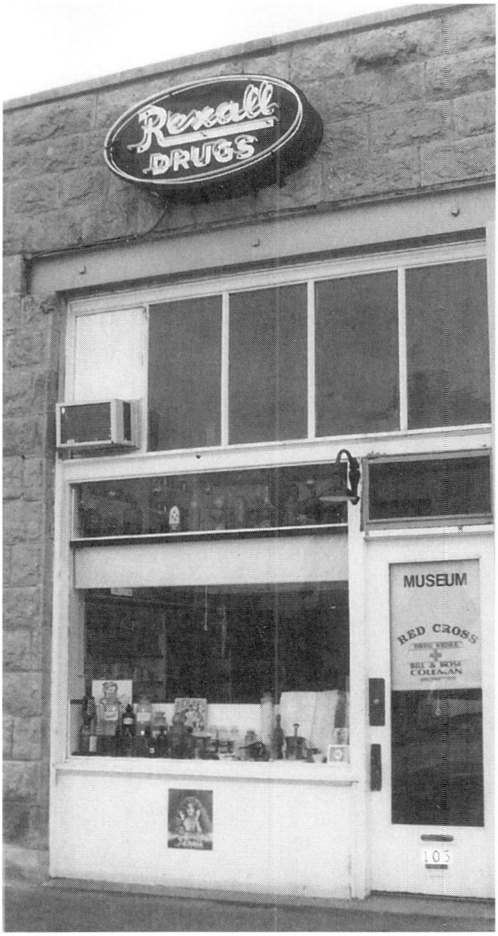

Red Cross Drugstore Museum
Wapato, Washington.

WEST VIRGINIA

MORGANTOWN

Cook-Hayman Pharmacy Museum
West Virginia University School of Pharmacy
Room 1132 RCB Health Science Center
Morgantown, WV 26506
(304) 293-5101

E-mail WRIDGWAY@WVU.EDU

Owned and operated by the West Virginia University School of Pharmacy. Art Jacknowitz and Clarke Ridgway, curators.

Monday - Friday 8:15 a.m. - 4:45 p.m.

Admission - fee for demonstration or group presentation (fee waived for educational groups).

The Cook-Hayman Pharmacy Museum houses a collection of mid- to late-nineteenth-century pharmacy artifacts. Included are botanical specimens, shelf jars, patent medicines, medicine bags, apothecary tools, books, pictures, almanacs, prescriptions, showglobes, cosmetics, and ephemera.

WISCONSIN

CASSVILLE

Wisconsin State Historical Society
Stonefield at the Nelson Dewey State Park Complex
Cassville, WI 53806
(608) 725-5210

Owned and operated by the Wisconsin State Historical Society. James Temmer, director.

May, June, September, October
Daily 10:00 a.m. - 4:00 p.m.
July and August
Daily 10:00 a.m. - 5:00 p.m.

Admission - adults \$6.50; students \$2.25.

This shop is part of a re-creation of a late-nineteenth-century Wisconsin village. It includes a pharmacy restoration of the late nineteenth and early twentieth centuries. Fixtures were moved from the Rydell Drug Store at Superior, Wisconsin. However, most of the artifacts came from the Rydell and Fred Mink Pharmacy in Cassville. Shelves are stocked with drug bottles and jars, as well as tools of the apothecary, and manufacturing equipment acquired from the defunct Willson-Monarch Laboratories. The exhibition also includes a cigar maker, confectionery and ice cream equipment, an 1890 pill-making machine, drug grinders, and mixers.

MADISON

Kremers Reference Files
American Institute of the History of Pharmacy
425 N. Charter Street
Madison, WI 53706
(608) 262-5378

E-mail krf@aihp.org

Owned and Operated by the American Institute of the History of Pharmacy and the University of Wisconsin School of Pharmacy Library. Gregory J. Higby, director.

Open weekdays by appointment.

Admission - free

The Kremers Reference Files contains a large number of reprints, tearsheets, illustrations, photographs and some manuscript material dealing with the development of drug standards. Originally collected for the purpose of writing a history of pharmacy (the resulting *Kremers and Urdang's History of Pharmacy*), the KRF occupies over 300 file cabinet drawers organized according to topical scheme. While strongest in the area of American pharmacy after 1880, the KRF holds historical material, primary and secondary, on almost all aspects of pharmacy. There are no artifacts on display. The Kremers Reference Files will be relocated to the new Pharmacy School - Rennebohm Hall, scheduled for Winter 2000.

Milwaukee

Milwaukee County Historical Center
910 North Third Street
Milwaukee, WI 53203
(414) 273-8288

Owned and operated by the Milwaukee County Historical Society. Harry H. Anderson, executive director.

Monday - Friday	9:30 a.m. - 5:00 p.m.
Saturday	10:00 a.m. - 5:00 p.m.
Sunday	1:00 p.m. - 5:00 p.m.

Admission - free

"Yesterday's Drugstore" represents pharmacy at the turn of the century. It features tools of the apothecary, counter scales, drug mills, apothecary jars, tinctures, cork and pill presses, mortars and pestles, a Diamond Dye cabinet, posters, mirrored prescription counter, show globes, a cash register, and patent medicines. The entire display was donated by the family of Theodore Marlewski, a Milwaukee pharmacist, after his death. The attractive custom-built fixtures were made in Milwaukee by a Polish cabinetmaker in the 1880s.

In addition, there is a physician's office of about 1900, which represents Dr. Nicholas Senn's (1844-1908) clinic. On display are an examining table, laboratory equipment, surgical instruments, sterilizing unit, diplomas and books, as well as medical kits, utensils, and remedies.

Milwaukee

Milwaukee Public Museum
800 West Wells Street
Milwaukee, WI 53233
(414) 278-2700

Owned by the County of Milwaukee. William Moynihan, director.

Daily	9:00 a.m. - 5:00 p.m.

Admission - adults $5.50; senior citizens $4.50; children $3.50.

This pharmacy replica along the museum's "Streets of Old Milwaukee" represents the period 1890-1910. On display are show globes, leech and gold-labeled drug jars, cobalt-blue bottles, patent medicines, shelfware and tools of the apothecary from several donations including the Otto Laab pharmacy fixtures and artifacts. Nearby is another exhibit of a period oculist's shop with tools and equipment, spectacles, and furnishings, illustrating some aspects of the history of American ophthalmology.

PRAIRIE DU CHIEN

Prairie du Chien Museum at Fort Crawford
717 S. Beaumont Road
Prairie du Chien, WI 53821
(608) 326-6960

Owned and operated by the Prairie du Chien Historical Society, Inc. Delores J. Igou, curator.

May 1 - October 31
Daily 10:00 a.m. - 5:00 p.m.

Admission - adults $2.50; senior citizens $2.00; children $1.00; families $6.00.

The Prairie du Chien Museum at Fort Crawford includes the reconstruction of a military hospital and a restoration of an 1880s pharmacy. The latter includes a prescription counter dating from the 1850s, and is complete with small glass peepholes through which the pharmacist could observe the front of the pharmacy while he was compounding prescriptions. Dioramas also illustrate the progress of surgery during the last century and tributes to both Dr. William Beaumont who performed the famous operation on the "man with a hole in his stomach," Alexis St. Martin; and Zachary Taylor, who was Fort Crawford's commandant when Dr. Beaumont joined the fort's military staff.

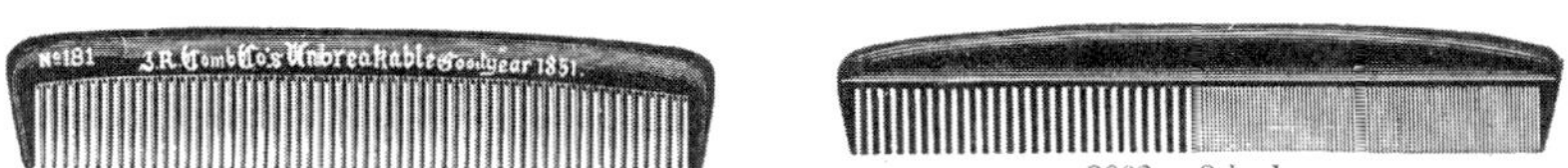

181. 8 inch. I. R. Unbreakable.

2002. 8 inch.

Pharmacy Museums and Historical Collections in Canada

ALBERTA

CALGARY

Heritage Park Historical Village
1900 Heritage Drive S.W.
Calgary, Alberta
T2V 2X3 Canada
(403) 255-1182

Owned by the City of Calgary and operated by the Heritage Park Society. R.R. Smith, general manager.

Victoria Day (late May) to June 30
Monday - Friday 10:00 a.m. - 4:00 p.m.
Saturday and Sunday 10:00 a.m. - 6:00 p.m.
July 1 to Labour Day
Daily 10:00 a.m. - 6:00 p.m.
Labour Day to Canadian Thanksgiving (US Columbus Day)
Saturday and Sunday 10:00 a.m. - 5:00 p.m.

Admission - adults $4.50; senior citizens and youth $3.25; children $2.00.

Heritage Park depicts life on the Canadian prairies from the fur trade era, through settlement of town and countryside until World War I. The pharmacy in the park was built originally in 1908 by F.E. Livingstone at Dundurn and subsequently relocated to Hanley, Saskatchewan. The interior boasts solid-oak fixtures ornamented with semi-Corinthian engraved pillars, a solid maple floor, and a ceiling of embossed tin. The pharmaceutical artifacts were collected for the project by the Alberta Pharmaceutical Association, Glenbow Museum, and Heritage Park.

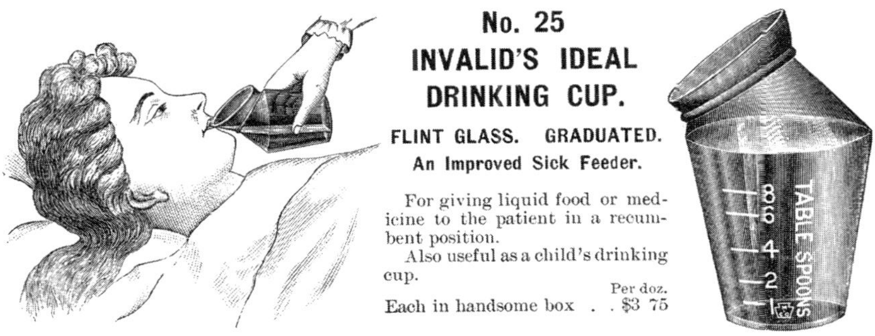

EDMONTON

Fort Edmonton Park
Fox Drive and Whitemud Drive
P.O. Box 2359
Edmonton, Alberta
T5J 2R7 Canada
(403) 496-8787

Website www.gov.edmonton.ab.ca/fort/

Owned and operated by the City of Edmonton. Brian Monaghan, director.

Victoria Day (late May) - Labour Day
Daily 10:00 a.m. - 6:00 p.m.
Sundays in September 10:00 a.m. - 6:00 p.m.
Call for Winter hours.

Admission - adults $6.75; senior citizens and students $5.00; children $3.25; families $20.00.

Daly's Drug Store re-creates a pharmacy typical of those in Edmonton in 1885. The drugstore combines the pharmacy with a dispensary, physicians office and residence. The practise was established originally in 1882, by Dr. H.C. Wilson, who had come from Ontario. He continued to practice medicine at the back of the premises until the 1890s, although he had sold the pharmacy in 1885 to Philip Daly of Fort Rouge, Manitoba. The professional practice aspects of the pharmacy have been re-created to represent the eclectic conditions that often prevailed in early pharmacies of the western frontier.

The Sun Drug Store was opened in 1920 by Sidney Millward. Mr. Millward graduated from the Faculty of Pharmacy at the University of Alberta in 1916. This was the first pharmacy university degree program offered in the British Empire. The Park's Sun Drug Store is currently interpreted on a volunteer basis by members of the Alberta Pharmaceutical Association.

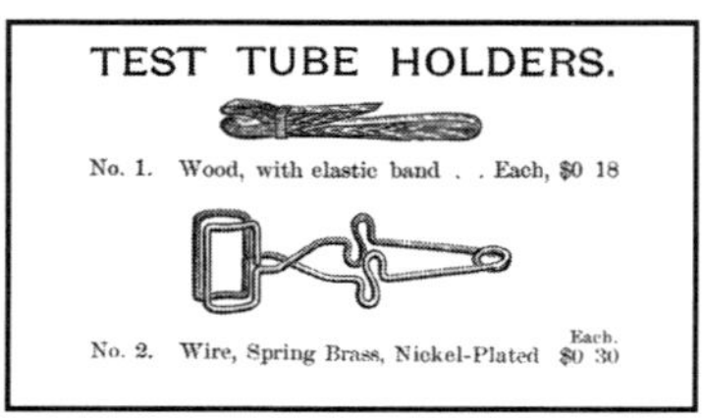

FORT McMURRAY

Heritage Park
King Street
Fort McMurray, Alberta
T9H 4H9 Canada
(403) 791-7575 (Heritage Park Office)

Operated by the Fort McMurray Historical Society. Kenneth R. L. Hill, director.

Summer Hours	
Monday - Friday	10:00 a.m. - 6:00 p.m.
Weekends	12:00 p.m. - 6:00 p.m.
Winter Hours	
Monday - Friday	8:30 a.m. - 4:30 p.m.

Admission - adults $2.00; senior citizens and students under 17 $1.00.

The Hill Drugs building in Heritage Park dates from 1934, since the frame structure built in 1921 was destroyed by fire and an earlier log building no longer exists. A modern Hill Drugs continues in the town proper, with a third generation Hill, as the longest operating business in Fort McMurray. Fort McMurray was originally the site where the railway ended and the river route northward began.

The 1934 building, moved to Heritage Park in 1965, houses a collection of artifacts and photographs which tell the story of the fur trade, the industries of fishing, lumbering, and boat building in the Fort McMurray area. It is the only building in the Park that contains displays, but no pharmaceutical artifacts.

BRITISH COLUMBIA

BARKERVILLE

Barkerville Historic Town
Box 19
Barkerville, British Columbia
V0K 1B0 Canada
(250) 994-3302

Owned and operated by the government of British Columbia, Ministry of Small Business, Tourism and Culture, Heritage Branch. Bill Quackenbush, curator.

Daily 8:30 a.m. - Dusk

Admission - call for fees.

Barkerville Historic Town celebrates the history of Northern British Columbia from the Gold Rush to the 1940s with an emphasis on the 1860 to 1890 period. There are twenty-two operating businesses, including a theatre and stage coach, as well as interpretation of domestic life, an 1870s school house, an operating water wheel, a blacksmith shop and early British Columbian justice. The Lee Chong Co. Chinese Museum celebrates the ethnic diversity of British Columbian history and the Caribou Museum that tells the story of mining for gold. There is an extensive archival research library that may be accessed by appointment.

The J.P. Taylor Drug Store, which operated during the early period of Barkerville's history, has been reconstructed with help from the South Vancouver Island Pharmacists' Association and the British Columbia Pharmaceutical Association. Most of the artifacts and fixtures came from the Thomas Shotbolt pharmacy in Victoria, one of the earliest pharmacies in the area. There is a collection of Shotbolt labels on display.

Burnaby

Burnaby Village Museum
6501 Deer Lake Avenue
Burnaby, British Columbia
V5G 3T6 Canada
(604) 293-6500

Operated by the Parks and Recreation Commission, City of Burnaby. Denis Nokony, manager cultural services.

May - September
Daily 11:00 a.m. - 4:30 p.m.

Admission - adults $6.35; children $3.80.

Finlayson's Pharmacy includes a general collection of pharmacy artifacts from the period 1890 - 1925, housed in a reconstructed building. The collection, gathered from pharmacies throughout British Columbia's lower mainland region, features apothecary globes, a set of rosewood herbal drawers, and Delft apothecary jars, as well as a wide range of glass storage bottles. A small archive is maintained containing prescription books and letter books from area pharmacies. The display was established with assistance from the University of British Columbia Faculty of Pharmaceutical Sciences and the Lower Mainland Pharmacists Association.

Way San Yuen Wat Kee and Company (Chinese herbalist's shop) consists of the entire contents of the shop which operated in Victoria from 1903 to 1970. It is set up in a reconstructed building to represent the pre-1926 period. It features a set of mahogany and rosewood herbal drawers with hand carving, a complete range of hand-manufacturing equipment, herb containers and many samples of old herbs and cures.

Fort Steele

Fort Steele Heritage Town
9851 Highway 93/95
Fort Steele, British Columbia
V0B 1N0 Canada
(250) 489-3351

Website www.fortsteele.bc.ca

Owned and operated by the Heritage Branch of the Ministry of Small Business, Tourism, and Culture of the Province of British Columbia. Derryll White, curator & archivist.

May to November
Daily — Dawn to Dusk

Admission - Call for fees

The pharmacy is a reconstruction of the Pioneer Drug Hall first opened in Fort Steele in 1896 by Arthur W. Bleasdell, who had come originally from Ontario. Artifacts and fixtures are also drawn from another early pharmacy located in Kimberley, British Columbia. The pharmacy is divided into a front shop and a dispensary at the rear.

Victoria

Royal British Columbia Museum
P.O. Box 9815
675 Belleville Street
Victoria, British Columbia
V8W 9W2 Canada
(250) 387-3706

Owned by the Province of British Columbia. J. R. Wardrop, manager.

Daily 9:00 a.m. - 5:00 p.m.

Admission - adults $7.00; senior citizens $3.21 and youth $2.14.

The L.G. Cook Pharmacy re-creates a shop circa 1900 and is situated with other similar establishments on a turn-of-the-century street in the museum's Modern History Gallery. Most of the pharmaceutical artifacts on display were donated by the British Columbia Pharmaceutical Association and installed by Bedford Bates, a local practising pharmacist. (The name of the pharmacy is taken from a fictitious character, since the streetscape is a composite, representative one.)

MANITOBA

Winnipeg

Manitoba Museum of Man and Nature
190 Rupert Avenue
Winnipeg, Manitoba
R3B 0N2 Canada
(204) 956-2830

Funded by the government of Manitoba, the Government of Canada, and corporate and individual support. George Wurtak, interim director.

Victoria Day to Labour Day
Daily 10:00 a.m. - 6:00 p.m.

Remainder of year

Tuesday - Friday	10:00 a.m. - 4:00 p.m.
Saturday, Sunday & Holidays	10:00 a.m. - 5:00 p.m.

Admission - adults $4.00; youth (4-17) and senior citizens $3.00.

Under the shop sign of "Bletcher & McDougall Drugs," this reconstruction represents pharmacy in a street of the 1920s. In addition to the customary front shop and dispensary stocked with such items as period drugs, proprietaries, and sundries, there is a small post office, and an area for the manufacture of pharmaceutical preparations. Cameras and photographic equipment are prominent among the artifacts on display. A typical embossed metal ceiling completes the picture. The project was carried out with the consultation and active participation of pharmacist C.G. Chapman and a committee of the Manitoba Pharmaceutical Association.

NEWFOUNDLAND

ST. JOHN'S

James J. O'Mara Pharmacy Museum
Apothecary Hall
488 Walter Street
St. John's, Newfoundland
A1E 1B3 Canada
(709) 753-5877

E-mail npha@nf.sympatico.ca

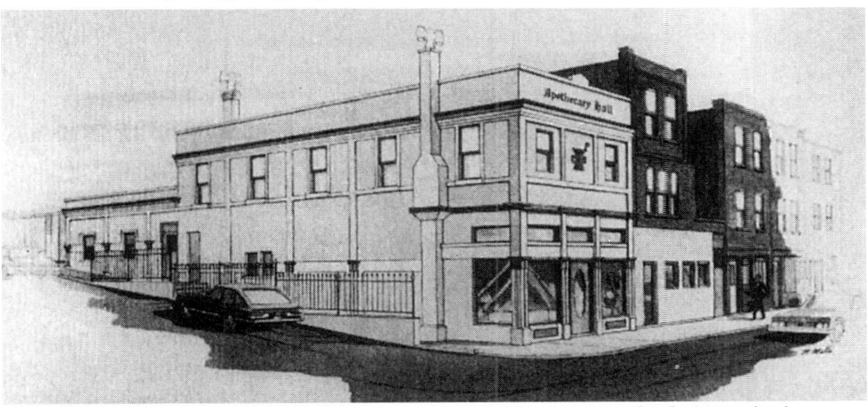

Apothecary Hall run by the Newfoundland Pharmaceutical Association.

Owned by the Newfoundland Pharmaceutical Association/Apothecary Hall Trust. Donald F. Rowe, secretary-registrar.

Mid-June - end of August 10:00 a.m. - 5:00 p.m.
By appointment rest of the year.

Admission - free

The museum contains approximately 1,500 items relating to the history of the association and pharmacy in Newfoundland. Included are books, artifacts, records, and proprietary remedies. Fixtures from the M. Connors pharmacy of St. John's, originally brought from England in 1879, have been incorporated into the re-creation of a pharmacy of the 1890s, complete with tin-embossed ceiling.

NOVA SCOTIA

GRANVILLE FERRY

The Habitation
Port Royal National Historic Park
Annapolis County
Granville Ferry, Nova Scotia
B0S 1K0 Canada
(902) 532-2397

Owned by Parks Canada, the Department of the Environment, the Government of Canada. J. D. How, area interpretive officer.

May 15 - June 15
Daily 9:00 a.m. - 5:00 p.m.
June 15 - Labour Day
Daily 9:00 a.m. - 6:00 p.m.
Labour Day - October 15
Daily 9:00 a.m. - 5:00 p.m.

Admission - free

The Habitation at Port Royal, founded in 1605, was the first permanent settlement in North America north of the Spanish settlement of Saint Augustine, Florida. Among those in the pioneering adventure was Louis Hébert, a Parisian apothecary, who thus became the first permanent pharmacist in the New World. He is also credited with being the first farmer in

Canada when he later settled at what is now Quebec City. The Habitation was reconstructed by the Canadian government in 1938 - 1939. In the room which Hébert apparently shared with the resident surgeon is a reproduction drug chest with drug jars and dried herbs of the period, along with other equipment.

SHERBROOKE

Sherbrooke Village
P.O. Box 285
Sherbrooke, Nova Scotia
B0J 3C0 Canada
(902) 522-2400 or 1-888 SHER-VIL

Operated by the Sherbrooke Restoration Commission. Craig MacDonald, director.

June 1- October 15 9:30 a.m. - 5:30 p.m.

Admission - adults $6.00; senior citizens $5.00; Children $3.00; Families $18.00.

The drug store is one of over 30 buildings restored to their original condition. The town was built on the site of a fur-trading post established in 1655 and prospered for many years as a lumbering and ship-building outlet. When gold was discovered in 1861, it enhanced the area's prominence. In this re-creation of a late nineteenth- to early twentieth-century pharmacy, period drugs, proprietary medicines, containers, and equipment are displayed. Demonstrations are also conducted throughout the season. Most of the artifacts were collected by the College of Pharmacy, Dalhousie University, while some of the fixtures came originally from Ontario. Professor J.G. Duff of the College of Pharmacy was the principal consultant for the project.

SYDNEY

The Jost House
54 Charlotte Street
Sydney, Nova Scotia
B1P 6W4 Canada
(902) 539-0366

Owned and operated by Old Sydney Society. Joan Young, administrator.

May 15- October 30
Monday - Saturday 10:00 a.m. - 4:00 p.m.

Admission - by donation.

The museum exhibits collections of local Cape Breton interest, which includes an apothecary that preserves an assortment of medicinals used in the early twentieth century. A display of apparatus and utensils used in the compounding of prescriptions also form part of this exhibit.

ONTARIO

DON MILLS (TORONTO)

History of Contraception Museum
19 Green Belt Drive
Don Mills, Ontario
M3C 1L9 Canada
(416) 382-5148

E-mail wmasanic@joica.jnj.com

Owned and operated by Janssen-Ortho, Inc. Walter C. Masanic, director.

Daily 9:00 a.m. - 3:30 p.m.

Admission - free

Eleven display cases featuring 625 contraceptive items from around the world.

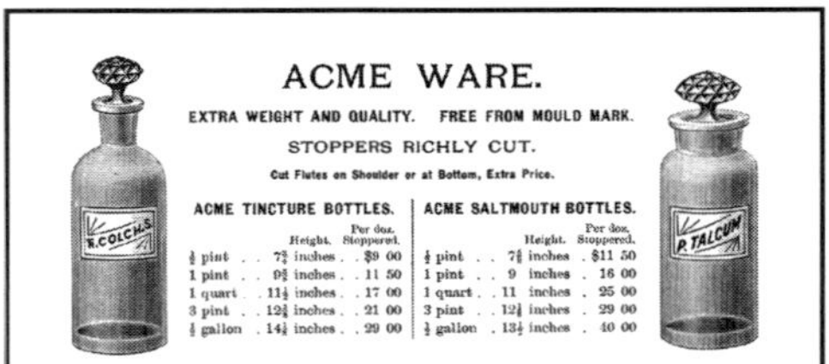

Lindsay

Victoria County Historical Museum
322 Kent Street West
Lindsay, Ontario
K9V 4Z1 Canada
(705) 324-6756

Owned and operated by Victoria County Historical Society. Lorraine Petzold, president.

Call for hours and admission fees.

The shop front, sign, and wall fixtures from the pharmacy operated in Cannington, Ontario, between 1907 and 1969 by G. B. Henderson, and prior to that, from the early 1870s by William and Simon Faed, form the basis of the Henderson Drug Store restoration. Many of the pharmacy's original artifacts, medicines, and herbal remedies are displayed.

Midland

Sainte-Marie Among the Hurons
Huronia Historical Parks
P.O. Box 160
Midland, Ontario
L4R 4K8 Canada
(705) 526-9193

Owned and operated by the Ministry of Tourism and Recreation, the government of the Province of Ontario. Rosemary Vyvyan, historical planner.

Victoria Day (late May) -Canadian Thanksgiving (US Columbus Day)
Daily 10:00 a.m. - 5:00 p.m.

Admission - adults $7.25; senior citizens and students $4.50; children (under 5) free.

Sainte-Marie was built in 1639 as the central residence of the Jesuit Mission to the Huron Indians. It was the only European settlement in Canada east of Quebec and Three Rivers. Saint-Marie was abandoned and destroyed by the missionaries in 1649 when adversities became insurmountable. It has now been reconstructed and an interpretive museum serves as its main entrance. A small extension of the hospital pharmacy has been restored and is stocked with purgatives and other herbs used for the treatment of colds and sore throats; some tools of the apothecary are also displayed in the museum. The shop is reputed to be the earliest pharmacy established in inland Canada and the northern United States. The apothecary, Joseph Molère, who was on duty in Sainte-Marie during the period of its existence, 1639-1649, also assisted the settlement's surgeon.

MINESING

Simcoe County Museum
R.R. 2
Minesing, Ontario
L0L 1Y0 Canada
(705) 728-3721

Owned and operated by the Corporation of the County of Simcoe. Gloria Taylor, curator.

Monday - Saturday	9:00 a.m. - 4:30 p.m.
Sunday	1:00 p.m. - 4:30 p.m.

Admission - adults $3.25; senior citizens $3.00; students $2.75; children $2.00; pre-schoolers, free.

The pharmacy re-creation is part of a village street of 1890 in the main building of the museum. Artifacts on display date from about 1870 to the turn of the century and have been collected from the area around Barrie.

NIAGARA-ON-THE-LAKE

Niagara Apothecary
Corner King and Queen Streets
P.O. Box 903
Niagara-on-the-Lake, Ontario
L0S 1J0 Canada
(905) 468-3845; off season (905) 962-4861

E-mail awlosek@ocpharma.com

Website www.ocpharma.com

Owned by the Ontario Heritage Foundation, Ministry of Citizenship, Culture and Recreation, the government of the Province of Ontario; operated by the Ontario College of Pharmacists. Ernst W. Stieb, curator.

Mid-May - Labour Day
Daily 12:00 p.m. - 6:00 p.m.

Admission - donations accepted.

This restoration, by Canada's foremost restoration architect, Peter Stokes, is a pharmacy that first opened on these premises in 1869; previously it had been at other locations in the town since the early nineteenth century. It is the only building surviving from this period in this historically and architecturally notable area. Fixtures are of black walnut and butternut and there are replicas of the original crystal chandeliers. Much of the original glass and ceramic ware, reputably imported from England about 1830, survives. Other artifacts date from about that period to about 1900. Original prescription and account records are from about 1830. Rotating exhibits from other collections are incorporated into the permanent collection of artifacts during each season. The mid-Victorian exterior is dominated by gracefully arched Florentine windows and a large gilt mortar-and-pestle shop sign. Closed as an active practice in 1964, little has changed since 1869.

SUTTON WEST

Georgina Village Museum
Civic Centre Road
P.O. Box 495
Sutton West, Ontario
L0E 1R0 Canada
(905) 476-4305

Owned and operated by Georgina Historical Society in conjunction with the Town of Georgina - Leisure services. Debbie Clymer, manager.

Mid-June - Labour Day
Tuesday - Sunday and holiday Mondays 10:00 a.m. - 5:00 p.m.

Admission - adults $3.00; senior citizens $2.00; children 6-18 $1.00.

Re-creation of an apothecary from the late 1800s in a village setting with a medicinal herb garden.

THUNDER BAY

Old Fort William
King Road
Vickers Heights P.O.
Thunder Bay, Ontario
P0T 2Z0 Canada
(807)473-2344

Website www.fortwilliam.on.ca

Owned and operated by the Ontario Ministry of Tourism. Elaine Nemeth, general manager.

Mid-May - mid October
Daily 9:00 a.m. - 5:00 p.m.

Admission - adults $10.00; senior citizens and students (13 and over) $8.00; students (6-12) $6.50; children 5 and under, free; family rate (of 4) $28.00.

Old Fort William is a living history site depicting the fur trade activities of the North West Company of Montréal in 1815. The Fort functioned as the Company's inland headquarters and transhipment point, and was the site of the annual Rendezvous each summer. The Fort features over 42-reconstructed buildings on a 25-acre site, situated beside the Kaminisitquia River. The site includes a working farm and active artisan trades. Although there are not many primary materials relating to the Fort's Apothecary, the Fort does possess material on Dr. John McLoughlin, one of the building's better known residents. Original artifacts, reproduction instruments, and chemical containers are on display.

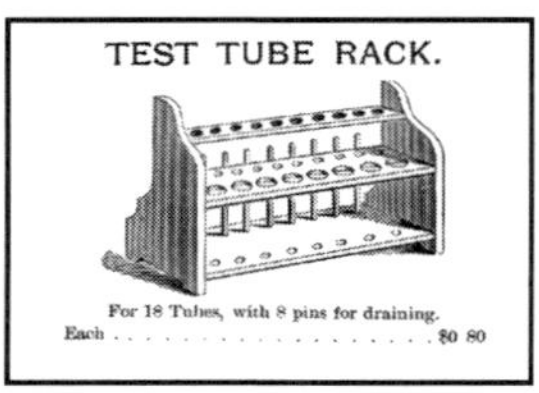

Toronto

Canadian Museum of Health and Medicine
Toronto Hospital, Bell Wing 1-651
585 University Avenue
Toronto, Ontario
M5G 2C4 Canada
(416) 340-4800 ext. 8557

E-mail Krumbold@torhosp.toronto.on.ca

Owned and operated by the University Health Network. Kathryn Rumbold, manager.

Call for hours.

The pharmacy and drug collection consists of some 2000 objects: equipment used for dispensing drugs (by both the pharmacist/apothecary and the doctor), pharmacy furnishings (both storage and decorative items), cased sets of prescription drugs, and patent medicines and their advertising material. The objects date from 1500 to the late twentieth century. The collection's strength lies in its European drug jars, dispensing pots, pill tiles and mortars. A small group of objects has a documented history of use by Ontario doctors, Ontario pharmacists, and Ontario residents. It dates from circa 1800 to 1920. The collection also includes drugs and furnishings from Chinese pharmaceutical practices in China and Indonesia.

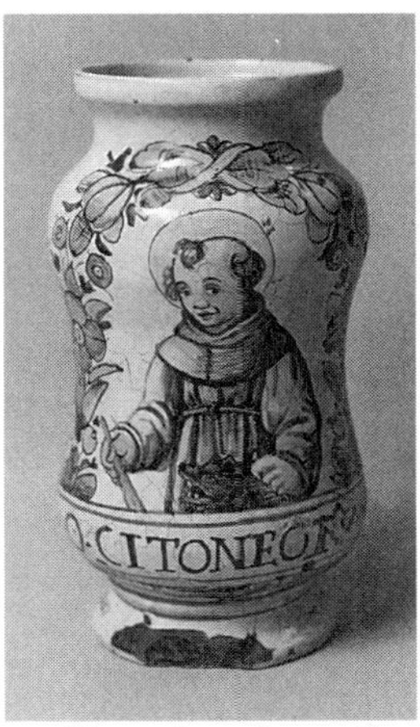

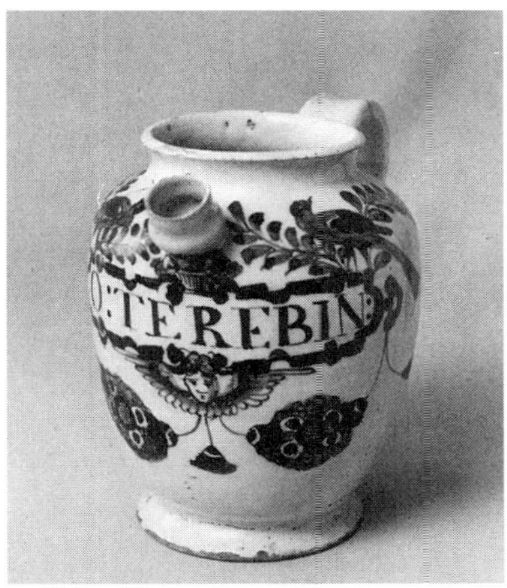

Drug jars from the collection of the Canadian Museum of Health and Medicine, Toronto, Ontario.

QUÉBEC

MONTRÉAL

Musée des Hospitalières
de l'Hôtel Dieu de Montréal
201, avenue des Pins Ouest
Montréal, Québec
H2W 1R5 Canada
(514) 849-2919

Governed by the Corporation du Musée des Hospitalières de l'Hôtel Dieu de Montréal. Sr. Thérèse Payer, director.

Mid June - Mid October
Tuesday - Friday 10:00 a.m. - 5:00 p.m.
Saturday and Sunday 1:00 p.m. - 5:00 p.m.
Mid October - Mid June
Wednesday - Sunday 1:00 p.m. - 5:00 p.m.

Admission - adults $5.00; senior citizens/students $3.00.

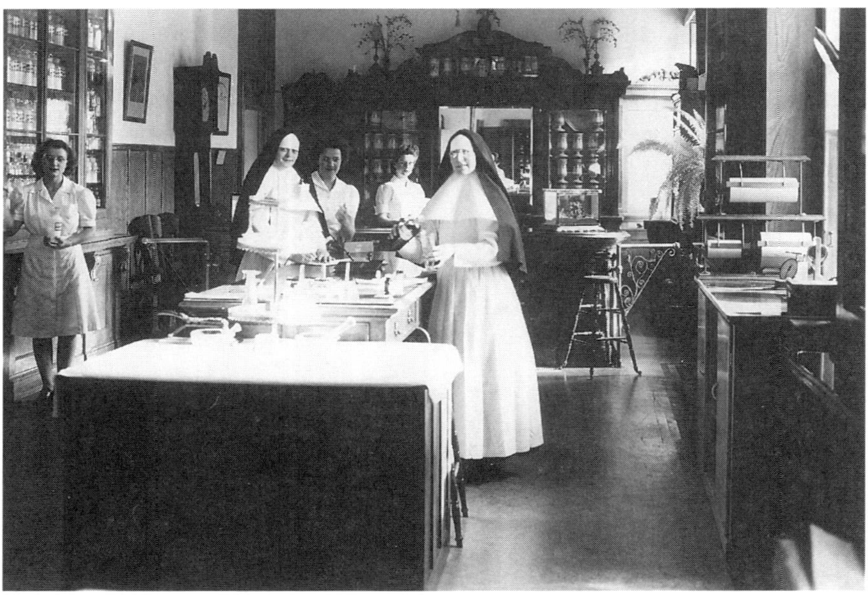

Pharmacie de l'Hôtel Dieu de Montréal, 1944.

The Musée des Hospitalières de l'Hôtel Dieu de Montréal on Pine Avenue traces the history of the Hospitallers of St. Joseph and their part in the founding of Montréal and Hôtel Dieu, the city's first hospital. The museum also provides a permanent home for a respectable artistic and historical collection, consisting of three and a half centuries of original drawings, paintings, letters, books, furniture, utensils and other objects pertaining to pharmacy.

Québec City

Monastére des Augustines
L'Hôpital Général de Québec
(Quebec General Hospital)
250 Boulevard Langelier
Québec City, Québec
G1K 5N1 Canada
(418) 529-0931

Owned and operated by the Soeurs Augustines de la Miséricorde de Jésus. Soeur Rita Caron, AMJ, responsable du musée.

Open to visitors by prior telephone appointment.

Admission - free

The hospital was founded in 1693 by Monseigneur St. Vallier, the second bishop of Québec, while the museum was opened between 1935 and 1940. The museum houses some notable artifacts, but most important is a superb collection of drug jars dating from the middle of the eighteenth-century. Sister Cloutier points out an important historic fact: "fire has never touched our walls, come see and you will marvel at what these old walls contain." She is also proud to point out that the museum is a private one, the property of the Monastery of the Augustines of the Mercy of Jesus, which receives no government subsidy. Some working knowledge of French or a French/English speaking companion or guide are recommended.

QUÉBEC CITY

Musée des Augustines
(Museum of the Hotel-Dieu Hospital)
75 rue des Remparts or 32 rue Charlevoix
Québec City, Québec
GIR 5C4 Canada
(418) 692-2492

Owned and operated by the Soeurs Augustines de la Miséricorde de Jesus. Nicole Perron, curator.

Tuesday - Saturday	9:30 a.m. - 12:00 p.m.
	1:30 p.m. - 5:00 p.m.
Sunday	1:30 p.m. - 5:00 p.m.

Admission - suggested donation $2.00 per person.

A remarkable, if somewhat disparate, collection of such things as medical and pharmaceutical equipment and containers, photographs, and manuscripts, dating back to 1639, when the hospital was first established. It is the oldest hospital in North America and one of the oldest in the British Commonwealth. When circumstances permit, visitors are also shown some of the oldest extant sections of the building. Some captions are bilingual, a bilingual catalog is available, and a bilingual guide is present at festival time, but a passable working knowledge of French may be desirable.

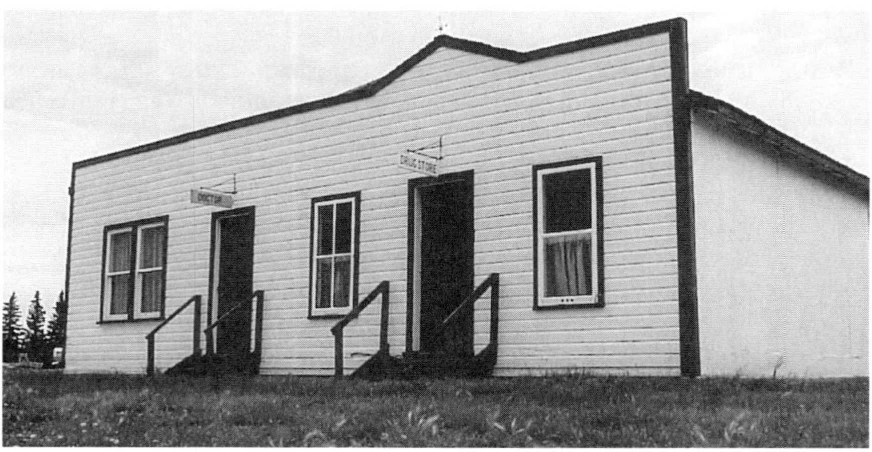

Drug Store exterior, Western Development Museum - Pioneer Village.

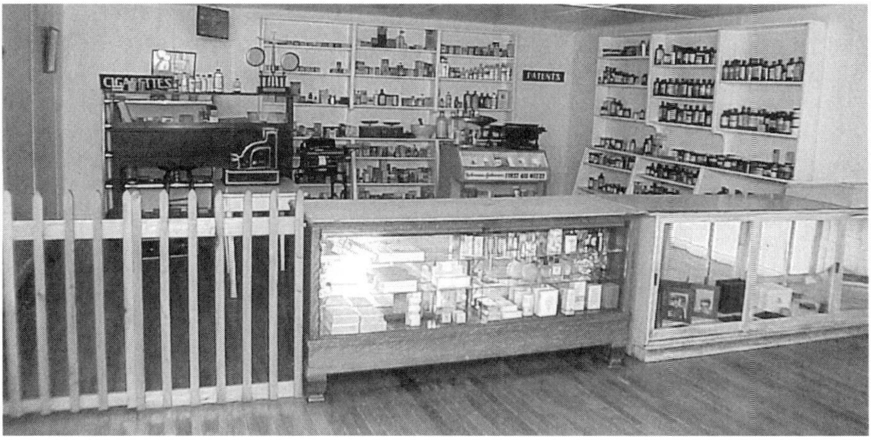

Interior of Drug Store, Western Development Museum -Pioneer Village.

SASKATCHEWAN

North Battleford

Western Development Museum and Pioneer Village
Box 183
North Battleford, Saskatchewan
S9A 2P1 Canada
(306) 445-8033

E-mail swdm@sk.sympatico.ca

Operated by the Saskatchewan Western Development Museum Board. R. Wayne Fennig, branch manager.

May 1 - October 15
Daily 9:00 a.m. - 7:00 p.m.
October 15 - April 30
Wednesday-Sunday 1:00 p.m. - 5:00 p.m.

Admission - adults $4.50; senior citizens/students $3.50; children $1.50; pre-schoolers free; families $12.00.

The North Battleford Heritage Museum & Village features a village and farmstead offering a glimpse of Saskatchewan life during the 1920s.

One of the outdoor village buildings is a doctor's office with waiting room, examination room and office. A drugstore representing the 1920s is a part of the village. Artifacts representing the profession include mortars and pestles, scales and balances, glassware, and compression device to make pills. Other items sold by the drugstore included veterinary supplies, stationery, grooming aids and toiletries.

REGINA

Saskatchewan Pharmacy Museum Society
700-4010 Pasqua Street
Regina, Saskatchewan
S4S 7B9 Canada
(306) 584-2292

E-mail saskpharm@sk.sympatico.ca

Owned and operated by the Saskatchewan Pharmacy Museum Society.

Monday - Friday	8:00 a.m. - 12:00 p.m. 1:00 p.m. - 4:30 p.m.

Admission - free

Pharmacy artifacts are collected throughout the province.

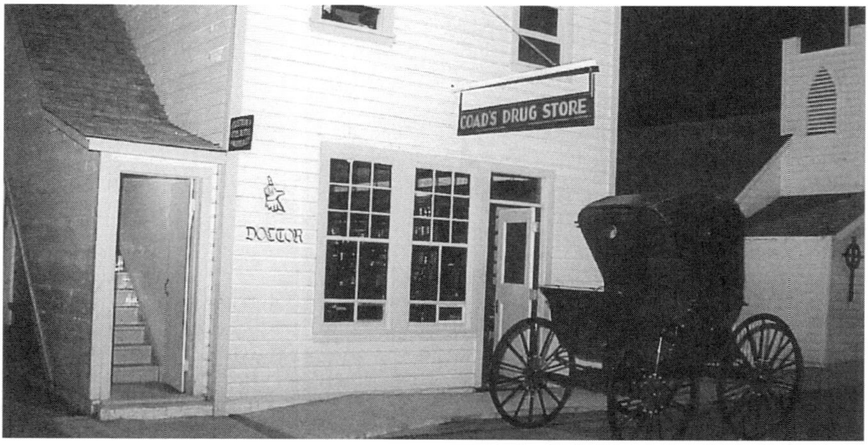

Coad's Drug Store - Western Development Museum - 1910 Boomtown.

SASKATOON

Saskatchewan Western Development Museum
1910 Boomtown
2610 Lorne Avenue
Saskatoon, Saskatchewan
S7K 0S6 Canada
(306) 931-1910

E-mail swdm@sk.sympatico.ca

Operated by the Saskatchewan Western Development Museum Board of Directors. Tom Waiser, manager, 1910 Boomtown.

Daily 9:00 a.m. - 5:00 p.m.

Admission - adults $4.50; senior citizens and students $3.50; children $1.50; pre-schoolers free; families $12.00.

1910 Boomtown is a representation of an early Saskatchewan town. Over 30 buildings portray community life during the bustling settlement period. One of the buildings featured is Coad's Drug Store, furnished with much of the equipment of an early Saskatoon drugstore. The original store was built about 1906. Included on display are dispensing artifacts, bottles, containers, prescription records and patent medicines.

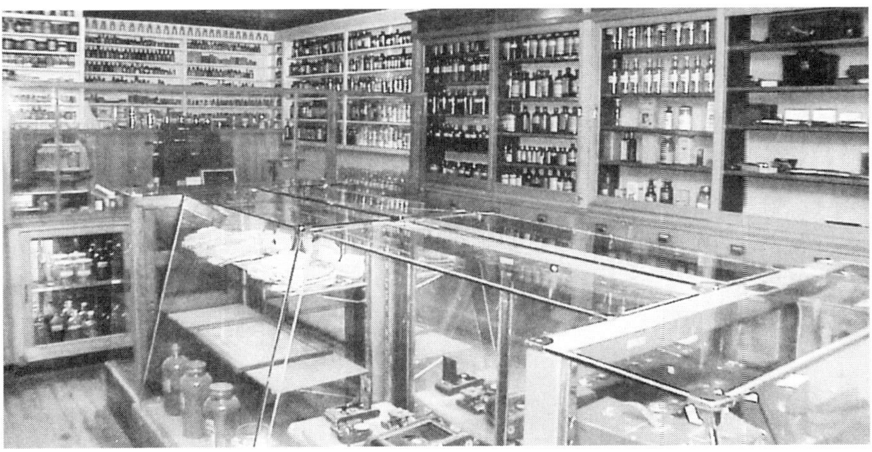

Interior Coad's Drug Store 1910 Boomtown
Western Development Museum, Saskatoon, Saskatchewan.

Historical Pharmacy Markers

A need to recognize noteworthy sites relating to important events in pharmaceutical history in the United States has been felt for over two decades. Historical markers placed at such sites would serve as reminders of some of the contributions that the profession, the pharmaceutical industry, and pharmacy's educational institutions have made to public health and welfare. Toward achieving this end, a committee in historical markers was formed during the 1958 annual meeting of the American Institute of the History of Pharmacy.

In 1959, the Institute's Council adopted a recommendation by this committee to implement a project "to mark and permanently recognize historical sites meaningful to American Pharmacy." Procedural outlines for implementing the program were prepared, and pharmacists and pharmaceutical organizations were encouraged to recommend specific sites for historical markers, to be reviewed by a committee and approved by the Council.[1] The first such site was marked three years later, in 1963.

The following is an annotated list of markers dedicated by the American Institute of the History of Pharmacy at historical sites for 1963 through 1999.

1. October 10, 1963: Site of the Pharmacy of Louis Joseph Dufilho, at 514 Chartres Street, New Orleans, Louisiana-in the heart of the old French Quarter-and known as La Pharmacie Francaise. Pharmacist Dufilho is recognized as one of the first pharmacists to be licensed in the United States. The plaque mounted just to the right of the doorway gives permanent recognition to pharmacy's vital significance of the improvement of public health. It symbolizes the beginning (1816) of a system of certifying professional competence of pharmacists in the United States, establishing an important principle by which the profession would eventually be recognized and regulated.[2] On this historical site, a pharmacy museum, one of the finest showcases of its kind in the country, was reconstituted and is open to the public (for description see pp. 38-39).

2. October 2, 1964; Site of founding of the American Pharmaceutical Association in Philadelphia, Pennsylvania, October 7, 1852. The plaque was placed in a stone column to the left of the main entrance of the Lit Brothers Department Store, located at 8th (near Filbert, then 710 Zane) and Market streets in the heart of downtown Philadelphia. Here was the original building of the Philadelphia College of Pharmacy where the Ameri-

can Pharmaceutical Association, the first and principal national professional society of pharmacists in this country, was founded.[3] The marker was removed during remodeling of the building in 1980, and plans for its replacement are currently uncertain.

3. January 22, 1966; Site of founding the American Institute of the History of Pharmacy on January 22, 1941. This event occurred in the old chemistry-pharmacy building (now Chamberlin Hall) at the University of Wisconsin at Madison (corner of University Avenue and Charter Street). It is stated on the plaque that the Institute was founded to help cultivate pharmacy's role in the history of human civilization, and to promote the humanistic and aesthetic values of the profession.[4]

4. October 18, 1967: Founding site of the University of Michigan Department of Pharmacy, which was consequential as the first in a state university. The plaque, installed at the College of Pharmacy Building at Ann Arbor, Michigan, commemorates physician-chemist Albert B. Prescott's introduction of the state university's pharmaceutical curriculum which was authorized in 1868. The Department of Pharmacy became a School of Pharmacy in 1876. The pharmacy curriculum at Michigan pioneered bold new concepts that eventually transformed American pharmaceutical education. Michigan introduced extensive laboratory instruction coupled with basic science, making the academic study of pharmacy practically a full-time occupation.[5]

5. May 19, 1972: Founding site of the Rho Chi Society, the national honor society of pharmacy which was charted in 1922. The plaque was installed at the old chemistry-pharmacy building at the University of Michigan at Ann Arbor on the fiftieth anniversary of the society recognizes its contribution to the encouragement of scientific research and high educational standards in pharmacy in the United States.[6]

6. August 2, 1974: Founding site of the University of Wisconsin's School of Pharmacy at Madison in 1883. The plaque was placed on South Hall, the original home of the Department of Pharmacy. The marker recognizes the school's national influence and its pioneering role in establishing the first four-year baccalaureate as a professional degree in pharmacy-first awarded in 1895-and the first Ph.D. as a research degree in pharmaceutical specialties in the United States which was first awarded in 1902. Both programs were pioneered by pharmacist-educator Edward Kremers.[7]

7. January 24, 1976: Site of the establishment in 1778 of a manufacturing pharmacy and "issuing store" for the Revolutionary forces by Apothecary-General Andrew Craigie. The marker was placed on a stone boulder on the grounds of the Army War College, Carlisle, Pennsylvania.[8]

8. June 12, 1976: Founding site of the pharmacy of the Pennsylvania Hospital at Philadelphia, established in 1752 as the first hospital pharmacy in the thirteen colonies. The plaque was placed on the doorway to

the room in the historic Pine Building that served as a part of the pharmacy at its second location, from 1800-1927, which is presently the office of the hospital's president. The first appointed apothecary was Jonathan Roberts, followed in 1755 by John Morgan. Here medication were prepared daily as prescribed by the attending physicians, illustrating the need for professional pharmaceutical skills and services in providing adequate treatment and cures for the sick.[9]

9. July 10, 1976: Site of the compilation of the "Lititz Pharmacopoeia." The marker was placed at the entrance of the Brothers' House if the Moravian Church built in 1759, which was used from December 1777 to August 1778 as a hospital for the Continental troops during the Revolutionary War. The "Lititz Pharmacopoeia," for the use of the medical department of the army, was prepared by Physician-General William Brown at Lititz and published in Philadelphia in 1778. It was the first American formulary--a pioneer effort at the standardization of drug formulas in this country.[10]

10. September 5, 1980: Site of the Northern Regional Research Laboratory, United States Department of Agriculture, where key contributions were made to the development of large-scale penicillin production in the 1940s. These included the introduction of submerged culture fermentation, the use of precursors to produce more effective penicillin, and the discovery of a mold strain more productive of penicillin.

11. June, 1983: Site of the botanic garden established by the Trustees of the Georgia Colony during the 1730s. Aided by funds from the Worshipful Society of Apothecaries of London, the establishment of the Savannah garden is recognized as the first activity of organized pharmacy in America.[11]

12. June 25, 1992: Site of the Stabler-Leadbeater Apothecary Shop, Alexandria, Virginia founded in 1792 and operated at this site of 141 years. "The shop is a unique reminder of the period when manufacturing , wholesaling, and dispensing of medicines were combined as a single enterprise of pharmacists in urban centers."[12] (For description, see p. 99.)

1. *Pharmacy in History*, vol. 4(1959), pp. 58 and 72, and vol. 5 (1960), pp. 59-60.
2. *Ibid.*, vol. 8 (1966), pp. 79-81; or "Relexions sur une vielle pharmacie americaine," *Revue d'Histoire de la pharmacie*, vol. 52 (1964), pp. 107-108.
3. *Pharmacy in History*, vol. 9 (1967), pp. 14, 22-24.
4. *Ibid.*, pp. 45, 51.
5. *Ibid.*, vol. 10 (1968), pp. 14-15.
6. *Ibid.*, vol. 14 (1972), 116-117.
7. *Ibid.*, 16 (1974), pp. 159-160.
8. *Ibid.*, vol. 18 (1976), pp. 69-71.
9. *Ibid.*, vol. 19 (1977), pp. 50-53.
10. *Ibid.*
11. *Ibid.*, vol. 26 (1984), pp. 40-41.
12. *Ibid.*, vol. 34 (1992), pp.193-194.

Name Index

The American Institute of the History of Pharmacy is a non-profit national organization devoted to advancing knowledge and understanding of the place of pharmacy in history.

Please join us and share in the exploration and preservation of pharmacy's heritage. All our programs are funded entirely by the contributions of past and present members. In return for your membership support you will receive yearly:

Pharmacy in History, the Institute's journal

a historical pharmacy calendar

booklets for the historian and general reader

textbooks, bibliographies, slide talks, and other materials at a 40% discount

For additional information contact:
American Institute of the History of Pharmacy
Pharmacy Building
University of Wisconsin
Madison, WI 53706
608-262-5378
membership@aihp.org
www.aihp.org